Advance Praise for

HOW TO NOURISH YOUR CHILD THROUGH AN EATING DISORDER

"A key tenet of family-based treatment (FBT) for adolescent anorexia nervosa (AN) is to empower parents so that *they* (the parents) can bring about weight restoration for their teen. This process is a delicate one—the clinician is to support the parents' efforts without telling them what to do, yet steering them in the right direction. Parents and providers can get tripped up in this task as weight restoration seldom follows a straight upward trajectory. A solid understanding of the nutritional requirements for recovery in AN is key to getting this task done. That said, the foundation model of FBT does not specify *how* best to integrate nutritional expertise in this treatment. This book offers a terrific start to this process—it will inform parents rather than prescribe to parents. Crosbie and Sterling take great care to use their nutritional expertise to complement the key FBT tenets. As a result, *How to Nourish Your Child Through an Eating Disorder* will be a helpful tool not only to parents, but also to the many clinicians who are tasked with supporting parents in their struggle to help their child overcome an eating disorder."

—**Daniel Le Grange, PhD,** Benioff UCSF Professor
in Children's Health and Eating Disorders director,
Department of Psychiatry and UCSF Weill Institute for Neurosciences,
University of California, San Francisco, and emeritus professor
of psychiatry and behavioral neuroscience, the University of Chicago

---

"For the parents of patients with eating disorders, this book, written by two prominent nutritionists, provides a comprehensive understanding of the illness and a practical approach to the refeeding process. Overall, an excellent summary of what parents need to know."

—**Martin Fisher, MD**, chief, Division of Adolescent Medicine,
Cohen Children's Medical Center, Northwell Health

"I highly recommend this book to any parent whose child has an eating disorder! *How To Nourish Your Child Through an Eating Disorder* provides concrete tools—based in science—in a friendly, compassionate, and easy-to-understand way."

—**Jenni Schaefer**, bestselling author of *Life Without Ed*; *Goodbye Ed, Hello Me*; and *Almost Anorexic*

"Parents: This book is your play-by-play for *exactly* how you can help your child heal their mind and body with food!"

—**Rebecca Scritchfield, RDN, EP-C**, author of *Body Kindness*

"Casey Crosbie and Wendy Sterling's practical book is an innovative and user-friendly resource on how to nourish a child with an eating disorder back to health. Crosbie and Sterling provide an important adjunctive approach to FBT, the first-line outpatient treatment for eating disorders. This excellent resource offers helpful strategies to empower parents and caregivers to play an active role in their adolescent's recovery."

—**Debra K. Katzman, MD, FRCPC**, professor of pediatrics, the Hospital for Sick Children and University of Toronto, and director of health science research, University of Toronto MD Program

---

"Family-based treatment is extremely effective, yet difficult. *How to Nourish Your Child Through an Eating Disorder* provides just the help parents need to ensure their child will recover at home."

—**Marcia Herrin, EdD, MPH, RDN, FAED**, author of the *Parent's Guide to Eating Disorders* and *Nutrition Counseling in the Treatment of Eating Disorders*

"Offering necessary support to families and caregivers facing an eating disorder, this book will be a lifesaver. Casey Crosbie and Wendy Sterling offer clarity and specific guidance on *how* to navigate the three phases of FBT with their Plate-by-Plate approach. Feeding *any* child is a phenomenal task, and when facing ED it really does take a village—crucially, including a registered dietitian (RD). I'm thrilled to have this resource to share with families who are coaching with me through this journey."

—**Becky Henry, CPCC, ACC**, founder and president, Hope Network, LLC, Eating Disorder Caregiver Support

"Providing relief for parents and clinicians, Crosbie and Sterling not only guide you on how to put together balanced plates to aid in the restoration of health, but also cover such topics as medical stability, when to sit your child out from exercise, and what to do when your child's old clothes no longer fit. The approach shines in coaching parents on the ultimate pursuit of food freedom for their child—and it works."

—**Signe Darpinian, LMFT, CEDS-S**, president of San Francisco Bay Area iaedp chapter and coauthor of *No Weigh!! A Teen's Guide to Body Image, Food, and Emotional Wisdom*

"Crosbie and Sterling, registered dietitians and experts in the treatment of eating disorders, have created a comprehensive yet easy-to-follow guide that addresses both the nutritional and emotional aspects of recovery. The practical and user-friendly tips are sure to help any family navigate the various phases of reducing fear and forming new and positive relationships with food."

—**Carrie Spindel Bashoff, PsyD**, child and adolescent clinical psychologist, adjunct assistant professor NYU School of Medicine

---

"Some of us are adrift in a fog of uncertainty at each meal we prepare. This book gives answers without tying us up in rules. Add this to your family-based treatment library for clear, competent guidance on food, exercise, weight, and health—and on what to serve to rebuild your child's flexibility, normalize their attitude toward eating, and prepare them for independence."

—**Eva Musby**, parent and author of *Anorexia and Other Eating Disorders: How to Help Your Child Eat Well and Be Well*

"This book is a must read for any parent with a child struggling with an unbalanced relationship with food. Wendy and Casey have developed a straightforward approach that equips and empowers parents to feed their child and achieve greater food freedom. They illustrate how parents can challenge fear foods through exposures, reduce obsessiveness related to food, and facilitate a more wholesome relationship to food, supporting a child's recovery through every step!"

—**Riley Nickols, PhD**, sport psychologist and director of the Victory Program

---

"An essential resource for parents of children struggling to overcome an eating disorder. This book boils down the science of eating disorder recovery with practical tips for every stage of healing. I wish my parents had access to this book when I was going through my eating disorder."

—**Kristina Saffran**, cofounder and CEO, Project HEAL

"When I was suffering with an eating disorder my parents struggled to find a book that could provide support and strategies both for themselves and for me. Today's parents are lucky to have *How to Nourish Your Child Through an Eating Disorder*, which provides great insight into how to effectively nourish your child at home through the innovative Plate-by-Plate approach. It's sure to help countless families!"

—**Liana Rosenman**, cofounder of Project HEAL

"With this invaluable resource, leading nutritionists Crosbie and Sterling coach parents on how to feed their child balanced meals using the Plate-by-Plate approach, helping them navigate the complex demands of the eating disorder—and empowering them to fight back."

—**Laura Kimeldorf, MD**, psychiatrist, New York City

"Food morphs into a crippling fear when an eating disorder develops. This Plate-by-Plate approach offers a way for parents and other caregivers to guide their loved one to dismantling the fear—and help renourish their mind and body and get their life back on track. I wish this had been available to my parents when I was a kid."

—**June Alexander, PhD,** author of *Using Writing as a Therapy for Eating Disorders* and coauthor with Daniel Le Grange of *My Kid Is Back*

How to Nourish Your Child Through an Eating Disorder

How to Nourish Your Child Through an Eating Disorder

A Simple, Plate-by-Plate Approach to Rebuilding a Healthy Relationship with Food

Casey Crosbie, RD, CSSD, and
Wendy Sterling, MS, RD, CSSD

Forewords by James Lock, MD, PhD,
and Neville H. Golden, MD

THE EXPERIMENT

NEW YORK

The Experiment, LLC
220 East 23rd Street, Suite 600
New York, NY 10010-4658
theexperimentpublishing.com

Library of Congress Cataloging-in-Publication Data

Names: Crosbie, Casey, author. | Sterling, Wendy, author.
Title: How to nourish your child through an eating disorder : a simple,
  plate-by-plate approach to rebuilding a healthy relationship with food /
  Casey Crosbie, RD, CSSD and Wendy Sterling, MS, RD, CSSD.
Description: New York : The Experiment, [2018] | Includes bibliographical
  references and index.
Identifiers: LCCN 2018005373 (print) | LCCN 2018007597 (ebook) | ISBN
  9781615194513 (Ebook) | ISBN 9781615194506 (pbk.)
Subjects: LCSH: Eating disorders in children. | Eating disorders in
  children--Patients--Family relationships. | Children--Nutrition. | Chronic
  diseases in children--Nutritional aspects.
Classification: LCC RJ506.E18 (ebook) | LCC RJ506.E18 C76 2018 (print) | DDC
  618.92/8526--dc23
LC record available at https://lccn.loc.gov/2018005373

ISBN 978-1-61519-450-6
Ebook ISBN 978-1-61519-451-3

Cover design by Sarah Schneider
Text design by Sophie Appel
Author photograph by Jenny Pfeiffer

Manufactured in the United States of America

First printing July 2018

10 9 8 7 6 5 4 3 2 1

CONTENTS

PART III: Returning to Normal

FOREWORD

O NLY TWO DECADES ago there were no evidence-based treatments for Anorexia Nervosa (AN), a disorder that had been first described in the medical literature in 1874. The common approach used until then was hospitalization for weight restoration plus individual therapy and family therapy aimed at developmental and family psychopathology. As Casey Crosbie and Wendy Sterling point out, things have changed. Instead of therapy aimed at changing psychological or family factors, family-based treatment (FBT) targets eating and other weight-loss behaviors that maintain low weight. FBT has emerged as an evidence-based, first line treatment recognized by treatment guidelines around the world.

The Plate-by-Plate approach introduced in *How to Nourish Your Child Through an Eating Disorder* uses the rationale and interventional structure of FBT as its basis. While the empirical support for FBT did not include the type of dietary consultation provided in this book, many parents using FBT have requested this assistance to help them be more successful in overcoming the behavioral challenges associated with their child's self-starvation and overexercise. Because FBT is fundamentally about *empowering* parents to make decisions themselves as how best to change these behaviors in their own homes and families, it requires a delicate balance when consulting about diet and activity. Trying to tell parents exactly what to do with strict rules on how to feed their child leads to many problems—including unproductive arguments over nutritional details and rigid rule following that ends up reinforcing eating-related preoccupations. On the other hand, not providing some guidance at times leaves parents feeling overwhelmed and uncertain about how best to proceed. This book succeeds by providing guidance for families to consider while promoting their own decision-making about what actually will work for their family and parenting style. It is my sincere hope that families find the guidance for improving nutrition in *How to Nourish Your Child Through an Eating Disorder* useful while implementing FBT with a licensed mental health provider. In this context, this book will prove to be the necessary dietary piece to help many families reach a lasting recovery.

James Lock, MD, PhD
Professor of Child Psychiatry and Pediatrics,
Stanford University School of Medicine
Director, Eating Disorder Program,
Lucile Packard Children's Hospital at Stanford

FOREWORD

WHEN A CHILD develops an eating disorder the family is suddenly thrust into a state of fear and despair. Parents often wonder, how did this happen? Did I miss the medical signs of malnutrition in my child? Will my child have this condition for the rest of their life? What can I do to help?

Eating disorders are serious, potentially deadly conditions. They can disrupt the family, isolate the child or adolescent, and lead to complex medical issues, some of which can be life-threatening and require medical admission to a hospital. Most of the medical complications that children experience as a result of their eating disorder occur either as a result of malnutrition or because of behaviors such as self-induced vomiting or laxative use. Fortunately, effective treatment is available. Family-based treatment (FBT) is a first line treatment for adolescents with eating disorders that has been shown to be very effective, in conjunction with close medical monitoring to ensure medical stability. Even though FBT suggests that parents should rely on their intuition to accomplish refeeding, refeeding a child with an eating disorder is unlike anything you have ever been asked to do previously. In particular, research has shown that after periods of starvation, the amount of energy (calories) required to restore health far exceeds the amount required for maintenance under regular conditions. In addition, metabolic requirements of children and adolescents are higher than those of adults because of the additional energy requirements for normal growth and development.

It is not easy to get a teen with an eating disorder to eat against their will, particularly in a culture where so much emphasis is placed on the "thin ideal," and where media messages are in direct conflict with messages provided by the treatment team. Fortunately, this book by Casey Crosbie and Wendy Sterling provides guidance on how to do so, utilizing the principles of FBT. In an easy-to-understand visual format, the Plate-by Plate approach helps parents with the challenging task of refeeding their child struggling with an eating disorder. This innovative method is easy to understand, simple, and user-friendly (across all cultures and types of food). It provides a seamless transition back to normal eating, once ready to do so. In the pages of this book you will find practical advice on how to add variety to meals and what to do when your child still isn't gaining weight, despite everything you have tried. Also addressed in this book is how to let go of food fears, restore food flexibility, and reintroduce physical activity. This invaluable tool should be on the bookshelf of every parent of a teen recently diagnosed with an eating disorder.

Neville H. Golden, MD
Chief, Division of Adolescent Medicine,
The Marron and Mary Elizabeth Kendrick Professor of Pediatrics
Stanford University School of Medicine

INTRODUCTION

"My child will self-destruct if I order pizza for dinner."

"Nobody understands what we're dealing with."

"We need help and have no idea where to start."

IF YOU ARE reading this book you know the grip that an eating disorder can hold on a child and you may desperately want to know how to help set them free. Perhaps you have heard your child say they "feel fat" and noticed them cutting out many of the foods they used to like. They may suddenly have become picky and particular about what they eat and how it is prepared. There may have been moments that have alarmed you, like when your child burst into tears because you added butter to the green beans, or when you caught them secretly doing crunches in their bed because they have now become obsessed with getting six-pack abs. As a parent, you are your child's greatest hope at beating this deadly illness and you will need to arm yourself with all the tools you can to fight it. This book was created for you and is meant to be an extra set of helping hands in the face of an eating disorder.

Currently, there are seventy million people who suffer from eating disorders worldwide, and 90 percent of them are between the ages of twelve and twenty-five. Eating disorders, commonly thought to affect affluent, Caucasian females, are also becoming increasingly more common among males, transgender adolescents, ethnic or racial minorities, as well as in countries where eating disorders were not previously reported.[1] Eating disorders do not discriminate, and they affect people of all shapes and sizes, causing them to be frequently overlooked.

Parents, often directly involved in the task of helping their teens to eat normally again, feel overwhelmed and immobilized by this task. Should they start slowly or dive right in? Should they include their child in decisions surrounding food? Should they add more protein? More fats? As registered dietitians with nearly thirty years of combined experience treating eating disorders, we have developed an approach to addressing these questions that is unlike any other used in eating-disorder treatment.

Feeding a child with an eating disorder is likely the hardest thing you have ever had to do, and yet providing nourishment to your child is an essential first step before recovery from this disease is possible. The caloric requirements necessary to nourish a child with an eating disorder can be two to three times their baseline, and plating such volume at mealtime is not intuitive, even for the most nutritionally savvy parents. Because the nature of an eating disorder is restrictive, secretive, and explosive, the task of nourishing your child back to health, a process referred to as "refeeding," is anything but easy. You will need all the help you can get to fight the disease.

We liken an eating disorder to a "monster" dictating your child's every food decision. It is a powerful beast, a force to be reckoned with, and it will require the strength of your entire village to take it down. This book will teach you to challenge that monster; to stand up to its demand to eat brown rice instead of white, or plain chicken breast instead of steak. It will encourage you to reach out to the members of your "village" and ask for love, help, and support so that you can remain steadfast in the face of the eating disorder. Part of your village will be the treatment team you hire for your child. It will consist of medical providers, therapists, dietitians, and psychiatrists, among others, all working together with you on behalf of your child struggling with an eating disorder.

A New Approach

The Plate-by-Plate approach is designed for all adolescents recovering from anorexia nervosa, bulimia nervosa, avoidant/restrictive food intake disorder, other specified feeding or eating disorder, and binge eating disorder. We will discuss these diagnoses further in chapter 2. Our approach provides a visual guide to what your child's nutrition should look like and puts you in charge of all aspects of refeeding. This approach minimizes obsessiveness from the start by removing calorie counting, measuring, and meal plan exchanges from the meal-planning equation. Using just a dinner plate, you will learn how to put together balanced meals that best support your child's nutritional goals. Through the use of colorful photos of plated meals, you will gain a visual sense of volume and balance. This book will empower you to take charge of all meal preparation and food shopping, to plate full plates, avoid diet and light foods, and challenge your child with foods they used to like but have since cut out due to the demands of their eating disorder. Inherent in this philosophy is flexibility, with an emphasis on plating "what looks normal" rather than plating a certain number of calories—eventually allowing for a seamless transition to normal eating.

This approach is complementary to family-based treatment (FBT). FBT is the leading outpatient treatment for adolescents with eating disorders. It is designed to achieve weight restoration and restore the health of your teen in the least restrictive environment, by putting you in charge of food until your teen is able to resume normal eating. In this way, you are empowered to win the food battle in the service of saving your child's life; the more you win, the more the eating disorder loses. This sends the message to a child with an eating disorder that they are loved, need to get better, and that disordered eating behaviors will not be accommodated.

You are asked to not only plate enough volume on your child's plate but to also challenge the rules set by your child's eating disorder. You will be encouraged to plate a variety of foods at each meal, and to plate foods your child used to love before the onset of the eating disorder. Your child may have become fearful and scared of many foods that they used to love. Their diet may be much narrower than it used to be, and they are likely eating the same "safe" foods over and over again. Your child, who previously hated vegetables, may try to convince you that they "love salad now." They may say that the "other" food is too unhealthy or too processed, or that they are scared that "those types of foods" will make them fat. These fears are part of the eating disorder and need to be addressed during the process of healing.

For some families, health and "wholesome nutrition" can almost feel religious. As a family, you may avoid added sugars and have a preference for foods that are whole grain, unprocessed, made from scratch, and organic and locally grown. Some families may choose to eat a completely homemade diet; meaning nothing from a box or a store. Parents who may have worked hard to follow these guidelines in the past might feel protective of that, and may not be interested in working on adding in foods that go against these philosophies. However, maintaining strict rules around eating indirectly teaches your child to follow strict rules with food. An individual *without* an eating disorder can generally self-manage how and when they want to be more flexible. Though adamant about not having sugar at home, they might spontaneously decide to have a cookie that looked good at the store. But kids with eating disorders don't typically have that sense of spontaneity or flexibility. It has to be cultivated and learned. In a rule-based food environment, it becomes challenging to teach the child this very important aspect of normal eating.

We will lead you through the process of "exposure," which will encourage you to serve your child the very foods they are avoiding, in order to help reduce food fears. Sure, it would be *way easier* to just let your child eat the same thing every day. At least they're eating, right? Wrong. Being able to consume a variety of foods without fear is your child's ticket to normal eating, food freedom, and ultimately a lasting recovery. There will never be a right time to fight those fears, and waiting for the stars to align and your child to welcome new foods won't happen unless you challenge them now. And it's important to act fast; the earlier your child gets treatment, the shorter their illness will last.[2] The struggle that you and your child go through during this time will give your child the greatest chance to be truly free of their eating disorder.

How to Nourish Your Child Through an Eating Disorder

Parents Take Control

Our approach is different from the variety of nutrition approaches out there, which include calorie counting, food measuring, and dividing food intake into "exchanges." The exchanges are based on the system used by diabetics and is the most common method used in treatment facilities today. Using an exchange approach, the individual with an eating disorder is given an allotment of servings per food group that they can then "spend" as they wish. The goal of an exchange-based meal plan is that all foods can be converted into exchanges and are therefore included in a daily meal plan. However, this method is both complicated and limiting. A slice of pizza might be two servings of grains, one dairy, one vegetable, and one fat. The fact that a bagel equals four servings of grains may scare an individual so much so that they may choose never to eat one again. The exchange approach requires a lot of counting and tallying throughout the day, which can increase obsessiveness around food and hold individuals back from eating food that doesn't fit perfectly into their food-item checklist. Teens will often take charge of their own meal plan, shutting out parents and giving plenty of room for their eating disorder to manipulate how they are "spending" their exchanges. This can cause a wedge between the adolescent with an eating disorder and their parents, while allowing the eating disorder to stay alive. This is directly opposed to FBT and the philosophy of this book, where parents are asked to take an active role in recovery and to take charge of the food in order to help free their child from the eating disorder.

Feeding Your Child Visually with Just a Plate

In 2011 the United States Department of Agriculture (USDA) began to use a plate-model visual approach to educate the general public about nutrition. They moved away from counting servings and moved toward creating "healthy messages" when they created MyPlate, a visual infographic of how much of each food group we should be eating that replaced the food pyramid with which many of us grew up. Our Plate-by-Plate approach is similar to the USDA's MyPlate in the sense that it provides you with a visual representation of how much and what your child should eat. However, MyPlate does not provide a sufficient volume of food for adolescents with eating disorders who also require weight restoration. MyPlate does not come close to providing enough volume of food to accomplish the goals of refeeding, which can be roughly 1.5 to 2 times higher than the baseline requirements. It was designed for the general public, not adolescents recovering from an eating disorder.

Much has been written on what constitutes "recovery" from an eating disorder, and for the most part, we follow the general belief that recovery is normalized eating, weight restoration, resumption of menses, improved health status, as well as improved cognitions and behaviors. But recovery is also the many smaller victories along the way that only those familiar with eating disorders will recognize—the ability to eat out at a restaurant with ease and even joy, the birthday cake that is received with happiness instead of dread, the shopping trip that ends with a stop for ice cream instead of tears, and a random comment about appearance from a relative that is simply ignored.

This book will walk you through the early stages of initiating a new meal plan and then adjusting it, and eventually preparing for the transition back to normal eating. We will discuss how to be successful not only in the house but also when out of the house—traveling, at a friend's house, or in restaurants. We will ask you to be a fierce detective against any way in which the eating disorder might still be grasping your child. This will empower you to take back the dinner table, and it will guide you through the process of helping your child achieve a strong and lasting recovery.

A note about pronouns

Ninety percent of adolescents with eating disorders are girls, but boys and nonbinary or gender-fluid individuals are also affected; we use the gender-neutral construction "they" throughout the book to acknowledge this range.

A note about case examples

Throughout this book we refer to case examples taken directly from our work with our clients over the years. All names have been changed to protect their privacy.

PART I

Where to Begin

CHAPTER 1

Understanding Eating Disorders and the Obsession with Food

DIAGNOSES ARE HELPFUL for giving a name to what is going on with your child. They are helpful for research, where there is a need to classify and investigate specific subgroups, and they are helpful for clinicians, to categorize conditions similarly across the world. Eating disorders may involve eating too little (restriction), eating too much (binging), vomiting or excessive exercise after eating (purging), or all of the above. For some kids, there is dramatic and noticeable weight loss, and for others there is no change in weight but instead there are profound medical complications associated with their eating-disorder symptoms. A child with anorexia may eat very small yet balanced meals, another might decide to cut out meals altogether but still eat sweets such as candy or brownies. Another child may be excessively and compulsively exercising, while yet another hasn't exercised in months. One might say they were not "trying" to lose weight, it "just happened." However, in all of these cases, your child can end up in severe medical danger.

Eating disorders typically begin during adolescence. The *Diagnostic and Statistical Manual of Mental Disorders, Fifth Edition (DSM-5)*, a manual used by health professionals to diagnose mental disorders, lists anorexia nervosa (AN), bulimia nervosa (BN), avoidant/restrictive food intake disorder (ARFID), other specified feeding or eating disorder (OSFED), and binge eating disorder (BED).[1] However, teens with eating disorders don't always fit into one diagnostic box; instead, they can often exhibit characteristics across several different eating-disorder diagnoses.

Recognizing Eating Disorders

Eating disorders affect people of all sizes, races, ethnicities, and age groups. Anorexia nervosa was previously diagnosed when someone reached a very low weight, lost their menstrual cycle, had a distorted body image, and was fearful of gaining weight. The most recent definition of anorexia nervosa published in the *DSM-5* has removed the weight cutoff and the diagnosis can be made without regard of menstrual status. The newer diagnostic criteria are more inclusive, capturing those who are suffering regardless of weight. The criteria for bulimia nervosa was adjusted from binging and purging three times per week for three months, to binging and purging once per week for three months. These updated diagnostic criteria help to capture a greater number of individuals suffering with an eating disorder and shift the focus to behavioral and cognitive symptoms.

New to the *DSM-5* criteria for eating disorders is the addition of avoidant/restrictive food intake disorder. Those with ARFID typically do not have weight or body-image concerns but restrict their intake because of texture, taste, smell, or due to stress, anxiety, fear of choking, vomiting, or swallowing. Those with ARFID are picky, eating a limited number of foods, perhaps from specific places, prepared in specific ways. They may enjoy eating a burger, but from only one restaurant and not from others. They may never have tried certain fruits and vegetables, and may love desserts.

Also new to the *DSM-5* is the addition of binge eating disorder, which clinically defines what a binge is and recognizes the psychological distress that comes along with it. Interestingly, BED is more than three times more common than AN and BN, and approximately 40 percent of those with BED are male.[2]

Last, otherwise specified feeding or eating disorder refers to those who have significant distress around food and weight but who do not meet the full criteria for any of the other eating disorders. There may be a high prevalence of those with OSFED, since it captures behaviors from many types of eating disorders.

As we list characteristics that are associated with eating disorders and/or disordered eating, many may sound familiar. You will read about "odd eating behaviors," such as kids who use the wrong utensil to eat. Plenty of people might do this. For example, your son may insist he eat his yogurt with a fork—what's wrong with that? Maybe nothing. If he always ate yogurt that way, sure it might be odd, but it wouldn't necessarily be worrisome. But if he used to eat yogurt with a spoon and then one day started using a fork, you should be curious about that. Kids with eating disorders often have reasons, both conscious and subconscious, for engaging in certain behaviors or rules.

Case Example: Rachel

Rachel, in the height of her eating disorder, ate her cereal each morning with a fork, letting the milk escape so she didn't have to consume as many calories. If Rachel also started bursting into tears in front of the mirror, and then, shortly after, missed her menstrual period, her parents should be concerned. It's not any one, isolated behavior that is concerning, rather it's the changes in behavior that become worrisome and should set off the alarm bells.

Disordered eating is common. A study conducted by Cornell University found that 40 percent of male football players surveyed engaged in some sort of disordered eating behavior.[3] Studies show that 35 to 57 percent of adolescent girls engage in crash dieting, fasting, or self-induced vomiting, or take diet pills or laxatives. Overweight girls are more likely than normal-weight girls to engage in such extreme dieting.[4] Even among clearly non-overweight girls, over one-third report dieting.[5] Girls who diet frequently are twelve times as likely to binge as girls who don't diet.[6]

As an individual reduces their food intake and/or loses weight, whether healthy or not, there is an increase in obsessiveness with food and weight. In one classic study, researchers studied the effects of starvation and refeeding in healthy male volunteers who underwent six months of semi-starvation. As part of the study, they explored the effects of starvation on behavior, personality, psychological health, and eating patterns. During the semi-starvation phase, the caloric intake of each subject was drastically reduced—causing each participant to lose an average of 25 percent of their body weight. As a result, subjects became preoccupied with food, obsessive around eating/exercising, became socially withdrawn, depressed, more anxious, had trouble concentrating, and performed worse on standardized tests. They played more with their food, ate over longer periods of time to savor the taste, spent more time reading cookbooks and menus, and spent most of their day planning their food intake. This study highlights the powerful effects that calorie restriction and weight loss, in and of itself, can have on anyone, especially anyone experiencing an eating disorder, like potentially your child.[7] Luckily, with nutrition rehabilitation, many of these symptoms can be resolved.

Behavioral Signs

There are several common characteristics that are typically seen in eating disorders. Having done this work for decades, we are still seeing new behaviors each day. As a parent, you know your child's normal behaviors better than anyone and will sense when something is off. Trust that intuition. Does your child's behavior feel normal to you? Does it make you feel uncomfortable? Has there been a change in their weight? If your child is experiencing new behaviors that have you alarmed in any way, we suggest checking in with a health professional (medical doctor, therapist, or dietitian) as soon as possible. Ultimately, even if you aren't sure whether what you are observing is concerning, there is no downside to discussing your concerns with a health provider. The prognosis for fighting eating disorders is much better when caught early.[8] In the next few pages we present a list of several characteristics and behaviors that are commonly seen with eating disorders.

Increased interest in food and exercise

You might find that your child expresses a new interest in health and wellness. They may have heard something in health class, or watched a movie advocating for avoiding fast food or eating a vegetarian diet. Those experiences may motivate them to start making changes to their own diet. Initially, you may welcome these changes because, let's be honest, most teens do not always make great choices with their food intake or activity level. Your child might take up cooking, start watching food shows on TV, begin an exercise program, try out for a new sport, or become increasingly particular about their overall diet. Some of this can be a good thing; however, it becomes a problem when their interest turns into an obsession.

Sorting foods into good foods and bad foods

Often, we see that kids will categorize foods as "good" and "bad." "Good foods," also known as "safe foods," are typically foods a person considers to be "good" or "healthy." Examples of safe foods may be fruit, yogurt, vegetables, chicken breast, and fish (and will vary by person). Conversely, "bad foods," also known as "fear foods" are foods that feel "scary" to eat. A person may label a food as "fattening," "disgusting," "unhealthy," "gross," or "too high in sugar." Fear foods might include potato chips, hamburgers, ice cream, pizza, cookies, soda, and candy (and will also vary by person).

Increased focus on body weight and shape

Adolescence is characterized by emotional and physical growth. As your child goes through puberty and experiences rapid physical changes, you may hear them talking about their dissatisfaction with their new and, what may seem like, foreign body. Suddenly, they may be talking about "feeling fat" or "needing to lose weight." They might complain more about their thighs, their stomach, their butt, and their arms. You might hear them say they want to get "jacked" and "ripped" or have six-pack abs. Most kids talk about their bodies during this time. But someone with an eating disorder tends to obsess about it and frequently becomes emotionally distressed.

Body checking

A child with an eating disorder might "body check"—they repeatedly check parts of their body with which they are dissatisfied. Some kids constantly pinch their belly fat to see if it has increased, or try on many different pairs of jeans to feel which ones have gotten tighter. Kids who are body checking will frequently ask those around them, "Do I look fat?" And if they have access to a scale at home, they may check their weight several times a day. Parents may observe these behaviors or they may not, as they are often done in secret.

Body checking can increase anxiety, depression, and body dissatisfaction.[9] A goal of treatment is to assess how often these behaviors occur and to stop them from happening. Nothing positive comes out of body checking. It is often like rubbing salt in a wound, making the wound sting even more than it already does.

Weight loss

Typically, weight loss is a sign that your child has had a change in energy balance. Your child may be eating less, exercising more, or both. Weight loss is not recommended even for overweight children, as it can interrupt growth and development. Instead, the American Academy of Pediatrics recommends that kids looking to lose weight maintain their weight while growing, as a result "stretching lengthwise."[10] The child might instead be guided on how to alter their diet to prevent the acceleration of a disease state. However, "diets" can often take a life of their own and can be dangerous in growing children. Thirty-five percent of "normal dieters" progress to pathological dieting. Of those, 20 to 25 percent progress to partial- or full-syndrome eating disorders.[11] Research shows that the most common behavior that will lead to an eating disorder is dieting, and according to *Time* magazine, 80 percent of children have been on a diet before they reach fourth grade.[12] Losing too much weight might come with a series of medical complications (to be discussed further in chapter 4). The faster a child loses weight, and the more weight they lose, the more intense the preoccupation with dieting might be.

Loss of menstrual cycle

In girls, losing too much weight can alter their menstrual cycle. While common for athletes to skip their menstrual periods, it is not normal. If a person is burning more calories than they are consuming, even if only slightly out of balance, their periods may become irregular (also known as oligomenorrhea). The loss of three menstrual cycles or more is known as amenorrhea. The loss of one's menstrual cycle is a physiological sign that the body is out of balance and frequently occurs when someone has lost too much weight or when their caloric intake is insufficient.[13] Dieting alone can be enough to alter one's menstrual cycle, as the body lacks sufficient energy to support the body's systems and turns off nonessential functions like menstruation.

Obsessive thinking

Eating disorders are often characterized by obsessions and preoccupations with food, weight, and shape. Obsessive thinking worsens as a person loses weight. Lucinda, a sixteen-year-old female struggling with anorexia, perfectly captured what obsessive thinking can sound like:

> I feel like a virus has taken over my mind, and I need to be powered down. My mind is exploding with thoughts around food. How much butter do I use? Should I use butter spray? Should I switch to low-fat milk—no, make that fat-free milk,

err, almond milk? How much yogurt do I leave leftover in the container—if I leave some I will eat fewer calories. . . . Should I use honey in my tea, or milk? But that would add calories—make that plain tea only. Should I skip my gummy bear vitamins . . . they have calories . . . but also provide nutrients, okay, maybe better to switch to the non-gummy variety, but what if my parents catch on? How do I hide all of these rules?!

We've found that many parents do not even know the extent to which their child is suffering; the extent to which the obsessive thinking is rooted in a child's behavior is often hidden from parents out of embarrassment, shame, or to protect the eating disorder. A child with an eating disorder may count calories, track their meals on apps, and spend most of the day thinking about food, weight, or shape. Some will admit to feeling exhausted from constantly tracking calories. A boy we worked with described the burden of these obsessive thoughts by saying he felt like he was in prison. Here is a photo of a food journal documenting one girl's obsession with calories.

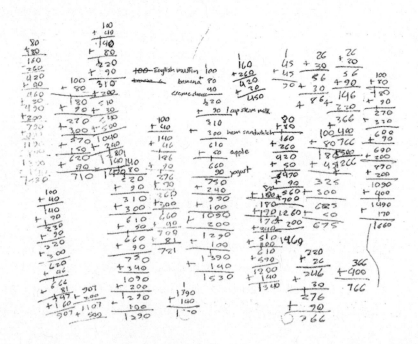

Obsessive thinking can turn into irrational and dangerous thinking. Heather told herself that she could only eat an apple and a banana each day, and if she was really hungry, she could eat a nonfat Greek yogurt. She followed that up by writing a note on her hand: *Apple. Banana. ONLY.* This behavior inevitably leads to heightened anxiety, as those suffering may or may not be able to stick with these often unattainable and dangerous goals. Someone suffering from an eating disorder may begin to talk about how many calories they need to burn in order to eat. "If I eat eight hundred calories today, then I have to burn eight hundred calories." This fails to capture the fact that your body is burning far more than what the treadmill might be reporting. The human body burns calories when digesting food (known as the thermic effect of food), during sleep, and also at rest.

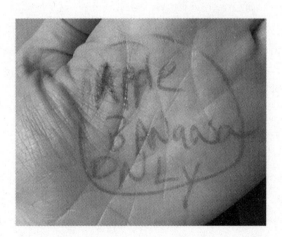

Increased rigidity and lack of spontaneity

Kids with eating disorders may develop new rules, such as "I won't eat after seven p.m." or "I will only eat what I can make myself." Some will have ritualistic eating practices, requiring meals to occur in a certain order, at a certain time, or with certain foods consumed first. Foods might not be allowed to touch on the plate. Kids who have strict guidelines for what they will or will not eat continue to be restrictive years later unless these behaviors are actively addressed. Those with eating disorders may struggle to eat in restaurants or attend basic social events like football games or concerts because "there is nothing for me to eat there." We have worked with kids who have packed measuring cups and a bathroom scale with them when traveling because they *need* these items, to be in control. This indicates the firm grasp the eating disorder holds over your child and suggests they are not ready to navigate the complex logistics that come with traveling (see Chapter 13: Eating on the Road for more details). We have also had kids who bring *their* food to birthday parties and other events. This immediately makes your child seem different and likely causes peers to catch on that something is wrong.

Normal eaters may grab a handful of chips or may take a bite of their parent's meal at dinner. As a child becomes more obsessive with dieting, their food spontaneity may vanish. They may be counting calories in their head, or just trying to eat as little as possible. Those who are following a meal plan may be fearful of eating outside of what they believe they *should* eat. Spontaneity does tend to come back in time as a person approaches true recovery.

Inability to try foods, outside of their meal plan

If you ordered a delicious entrée at a restaurant, would your child try a bite? How about if you go to the farmers' market, would your child try any food samples? Does it bother your child to take an extra bite of food outside of their set meals and snacks? You may have heard that it's not good to pick and graze on food throughout the day, but that is not what we are talking about. The ability to have a random bite of food, out of turn, is part of "normal" eating. This is the ability for your child to try Grandma's homemade soup when she offers a spoonful, rather than say no because it's only 4:00 p.m. and dinner isn't until 6:00 p.m.

Lack of spontaneity

Usually this is a big area of struggle for those suffering with eating disorders. All of these rules tend to hold kids back from being spontaneous.

If your child's friends are going out for ice cream after school, can they join them? What if they're going for ice cream at an odd time that they normally wouldn't expect to eat? Can your child join them anyway? The ability to be spontaneous is a gateway to freedom from rigidity around food.

Lack of variety

There may be a lack of variety in food choices at meals and snacks, not only throughout the day but also throughout the week. If you keep a seven-day food record, logging all meals and all snacks, how varied is your child's diet? Are they eating the same thing for breakfast most days? For snacks? Is the format of your child's meals the same? Limited consumption of food and food groups might intensify their fear of food and limit their ability to get a wide variety of nutrients.

Lack of flexibility

Due to firmly held beliefs around food or how food should be prepared, someone with an eating disorder may struggle to find something to eat when out of their home environment. We see this play out in restaurants, on the road, in college, when traveling, at a friend's house, at a birthday party, etc.

One of our clients refused to eat at In-N-Out Burger on the way home from his soccer game. "I would rather not eat than have fast food," he said at the time. But it was four hours later until he was able to eat at home. He missed the recovery window post-workout, which arguably would harm him more than having In-N-Out. In fact, many sports nutritionists would likely agree that given the choice between eating fast food or skipping the post-workout meal and eating nothing, it is better for you to eat fast food post-workout.

Someone with an eating disorder may only be comfortable with their own "special bread" from a specific health-food store or brown rice and not white. But flexibility around food is important. For example, if you run out of quinoa, can your child accept a change in their dinner for that night? Or if you go to a friend's or relative's house for dinner, and mashed potatoes are served, can your child eat it? If you find yourself catering to constant food rules set by your child, it is a sign that they may need help improving their food flexibility.

Kids may become so convinced that how they are eating is better than how everyone else is eating that they might look down on others and try to educate and correct them.

Avoidance of social situations

Your child may suddenly decide to skip social events such as a friend's barbecue or the school dance. They may avoid sleepovers, refuse to go to school, or opt to stay home instead of eating at a friend's house.

Compensatory behaviors

A compensatory behavior, defined as a behavior used to eliminate the calories consumed, is a hallmark feature of BN, but is also present in AN, BED, and OSFED. Compensatory behaviors can be vomiting after meals, excessive exercise, misuse of laxatives, diuretics, diet pills, and teas, or it can be a period of food restriction. Your kids may say, "I couldn't stop eating. I ate and ate until my stomach hurt. I knew I needed to get rid of it right away." "If I eat cake, I will exercise until I burn the three hundred and twenty calories that are in that piece of cake." "I had an extra scoop of rice, so after dinner, I did twenty-five sit-ups."

Strange and miscellaneous eating behaviors

There may be an unusual combination of foods consumed together, such as oatmeal with ketchup, or an excessive consumption of condiments and caffeine.

Case Example: Amanda

Amanda, a sixteen-year-old girl, began using Splenda in her coffee. She would put six packets of Splenda in a twenty-four-ounce cup of coffee, and would have three large cups a day. That's eighteen packets of sweetener per day, and at seven days a week, that adds up to 126 packets per week!

There might be an excessive use of salt, pepper, spices, soy sauce, balsamic vinegar, or hot sauce—spices and condiments that add flavor but don't add calories. Often in eating disorders, the body and mind are starved for calories and seek out a more intense flavor.[14]

You may notice your child making odd-looking meals that are not cohesive. Your child may mean well, putting meals together that have a variety of food groups. But they may fail to see the picture of the meal as a whole. An example of a meal that is not cohesive may be "bulgur, guacamole, a string cheese, and broccoli" or "one cup of miso soup, canned tuna, cereal, and blueberries." The items seem to be thrown together, some hot, some cold, and don't particularly complement each other. This may be partially due to an increase in food cravings during a state of starvation, or it could be related to the fact that they have entirely forgotten how to put meals together. It could also be due to having a very narrow range of acceptable foods, so there may be less from which to choose. You may also notice that your child may use the wrong utensil for the job, as in the earlier example of the child who eats cereal with a fork. Another example might be a kid using chopsticks to eat their cereal, or their old baby spoon to eat their soup.

Here is a list of commonly observed food behaviors exhibited by adolescents with eating disorders. These behaviors should raise a red flag.

- Cutting food into tiny pieces
- Ripping and pulling foods apart
- Eating slowly or taking small bites
- Excessive intake of fluids with meals or snacks
- Eating rapidly
- Organizing food on the plate before eating
- Eating foods in a specific order
- Letting food drop on the floor or table, or spilling beverages
- Hiding food (under dishes or napkins)
- Spitting food into napkins
- Excessive use of napkins, or wiping mouth, hands, or silverware on napkins excessively
- Constantly talking about food during the meal

Throughout the refeeding process, a process otherwise referred to as "nutritional rehabilitation," food choices improve and the obsessions about food decrease in frequency and intensity.[15] The best chance for reducing obsessiveness and preoccupation with food is for your child to achieve a balanced, healthy diet that meets their unique energy requirements. As a parent, you know your child best, and if you find yourself questioning the motives behind your child's newfound behaviors, by all means seek help. It is much easier to prevent an eating disorder from fully developing than to treat it once it's full-blown. Rely on your intuition. If something feels off to you, it probably is. Don't be scared to confront your child and to explore or discuss what you observe. The sooner you catch on to your child's eating disorder, the better the prognosis.

Orthorexia: An Intensified Focus on Health and Dieting

"I cut out gluten and dairy, I don't eat meat, I don't eat fried foods, I don't eat processed foods, and I definitely don't eat foods that have sugar." So, what *do* you eat? An extreme version of "health consciousness" has been called orthorexia, and is commonly (but not always) seen in those with eating disorders. Orthorexia, a term coined by Dr. Steven Bratman in his popular book *Health Food Junkies*, refers to an obsession with health and nutrition that becomes all-encompassing. Though not a formal eating-disorder diagnosis, orthorexia refers to those who have become excessively preoccupied with "eating healthy" and "eating clean," to the point that it disturbs the flow of one's life. Someone with orthorexia may have an eating disorder or may not, but they will likely exhibit many of the same behavioral signs seen in eating disorders, such as obsessive thinking and having a limited diet with rigid rules. With orthorexia there tends to be a focus on quality over quantity and on health over losing weight. Someone with orthorexia might be at a healthy weight and getting regular periods, yet they are excessively preoccupied with achieving "perfect" health. They might only choose foods that are free of additives, homemade, high in fiber, or low in sugar. And in a world of quinoa and zoodles, it's easy to blend in. But there is a difference between someone who has an allergy or a preference and someone who is hiding behind those things because they are scared to step out of their comfort zone.

With the influx of health messages, orthorexia has become increasingly common and can be debilitating. Kids who are looking to "become healthy" are attracted to this messaging, yet an extreme adherence to these messages can, ironically, cause kids to become unhealthy. Similar to traditional eating disorders, consequences of orthorexia include increased irritability, depression, anxiety, poor relationships with others, social avoidance, feelings of guilt, and an excessive amount of time spent thinking about or preparing meals, which takes time away from other activities. Here are some characteristics typically seen with orthorexia and/or eating disorders. Some kids may have one or two of these behaviors or beliefs around food, however in the case of orthorexia, a person usually exhibits most, if not all, of the behaviors.

Obsession with "health" and "eating clean"

Someone with orthorexia is obsessed with eating whatever is the most healthy and has difficulty deviating from that path under any circumstances. They may only eat brown rice and not white rice, or only eat organic, cage-free, grass-fed, free-range foods. They may prefer to bring their own bread with them when they go to lunch, predicting the restaurant may not have a "healthy enough" bread. They may spend an inordinate amount of time in farmers' markets, speaking directly to farmers to source their food.

Taking health messages to the extreme

As incidences of heart disease, diabetes, and cancer have risen, much of society is focused on diet and exercise, making the diet industry a fifty-billion-dollar-a-year enterprise.[16] Teens receive nutrition information from so many sources: school, friends, relatives, TV or internet ads, and social media, to name a few. Exaggerated and extreme responses to nutrition information are common in this population. There tends to be no moderation. If a high consumption of juices is associated with an increased risk of diabetes and obesity, then someone with orthorexia may stop drinking juice *forever*. Despite the fact that these messages may not be meant for growing and developing adolescents, teens hear them and apply them to themselves. In 2015 the World Health Organization found that eating processed meat can increase the risk of cancer; after that we saw numbers of kids with eating disorders swear off meat.

Particular requests and instructions for how food should be prepared

With eating disorders, and particularly with orthorexia, your child might have what seems like a million instructions for you or a waiter in a restaurant. "Steam the vegetables, put the sauce on the side, no bacon, no butter, a side of lemon, and please add three ice cubes in my water with a straw." Be honest. Does the family find it really annoying to eat in a restaurant with your child? Usually with orthorexia, a person may have specific food requests about what they want, how they want it prepared, and which ingredients to omit from their order. More often than not, they won't be able to even eat in a restaurant, becoming too fearful of how the restaurant is preparing the food and from where the restaurant is getting its meat and produce.

Does your child insist upon cooking their own food? Or being in the kitchen overlooking how you are cooking? Does your child complain that you are using too much oil? Too much cream? Adding too much cheese? Can your child attend Thanksgiving without bringing along their own food? Unless your child has a food allergy, bringing their own food is a sign that something is wrong.

Plain, dry food

Typically, those with eating disorders/othorexia eat a very plain diet. They will say it's "clean," but others may say it's "boring." A typical meal might be a plain breast of chicken, sweet potato, and a salad without dressing. There is no stir-fry sauce, seasoning, or flavor. Food is meant to be enjoyed; the combination of spices and flavors bring out the tastes of different ingredients in the dish. For some reason, those with orthorexia may think that sauces are unhealthy and should be avoided. Or that you should skip the salad dressing when eating salad. Really? That sounds like a torturous way to eat salad!

As you can see there are many different signs and symptoms associated with eating disorders and/or disordered eating that might be of concern to you. Some behaviors might feel benign, such as a newfound interest in health, and others might seem more concerning, like if your child is becoming more and more restricted and limited in what they will and will not eat. A progressively narrowing diet is always a concern for a growing teen, because it increases the likelihood that your child is not getting enough nutrition to support their growing body.

Our experience is that parents usually have a good intuition for when to be concerned. Talking about what you observe, naming it to your child, is a good first step in addressing what you see and identifying the behavior as a "concern." And don't be afraid to intervene—you can disallow your child to exercise at odd hours, or add in extra supervision if your child is constantly running to the bathroom after meals. You can begin the Plate-by-Plate approach—to be explained in this book in chapter 7—by making sure your child's plates are balanced and sufficient, even if your child hasn't been "fully" diagnosed with an eating disorder. This will help make sure your child is getting in enough food and prevent the negative medical consequences that can occur even from a small deficit of nutrition.

CHAPTER 2

——————◗

Family-Based Treatment (FBT)

By Nan Shaw, LCSW

————————————————————

IF **YOUR CHILD** has received the diagnosis of an eating disorder, the next step is seeking the best treatment. This chapter will outline the most extensively studied and vetted approach for treating eating disorders in adolescents, family-based treatment (FBT), where parents are asked to take over all aspects of meal planning and feeding. It is important to appreciate the dramatic shift that an eating disorder diagnosis, and then its treatment, creates for everyone in your family. Refeeding your child will, necessarily, become a priority above most aspects of life, including school, work, sports, and social functions. As you embrace FBT, you will commit, for now, to leaving regular life behind and becoming immersed in the treatment of your child's illness.

FBT changes the approach to food, requiring that you go beyond your child's historical food choices and the specific food requests that the eating disorder mandates. Think "food as medicine," with the primary goals being weight and health restoration. "Food as medicine" is the mantra in FBT. You'll use FBT in conjunction with the Plate-by-Plate approach, described in part II, which offers a simple way to understand appropriate "dosing" of this medicine—that is, how much food to serve your child.

As you embark on eating-disorder treatment, your whole family may suddenly find itself in strange and uncharted waters. You may start to realize that all that you thought you knew about "how to eat healthy" suddenly no longer applies to your child. This is common, and this book will give you the tools you need to navigate this challenging journey. FBT, together with the Plate-by-Plate approach, seeks to offer you clear direction and user-friendly tools to set you and your child on the course toward recovery.

Family-Based Treatment: Setting the Course

Recovery from an eating disorder is an active process, not a passive one, and has been shown to have the greatest chance of success if it can be handled with you, the parents, at the helm. In FBT, you will find yourself taking on new roles with your child and their food. You will become an expert in refeeding: supervising all meals, understanding your teen's medical vital signs, and figuring out how to put together calorically dense meals (meals high in calories). You'll also be setting expectations and limits. Helping your child get better specifically means no longer catering to the quirky choices that may have become the norm, with the goal of weight gain and normalized eating.

Initially, you may find yourself juggling "how we used to do things" or "how the eating disorder had tricked us into doing things" versus "what the family-based treatment requires we do now." In your quest to get your child to eat, you may feel that you'll do anything—that "something is better than nothing." We often hear families share compassionate, desperate narratives about their recent attempts to accommodate their child's food preferences. They are trying to find ways to make sugar-free pudding with avocados, or to create coherent meals out of increasingly smaller lists of acceptable or "safe" foods for their adolescent. But in the long run, "something" may not be "better than nothing" if it allows the eating disorder to stay in charge.

Where to Begin

At first, often parents report feeling stuck in their conflicting attempts to help their child to *feel* better (offering nonfat frozen yogurt) but also to help their child *get* better (requiring they eat regular ice cream). The central shift in mind-set at the heart of FBT is that getting better takes precedence over feeling better. In FBT, the belief is that helping your child *feel* better about food choices or amounts usually means the eating disorder is being appeased and the goal of recovery is being thwarted.

Many parents report that they have lost their limit-setting ability in the face of the eating disorder, and FBT seeks to help you find it again. While parents generally understand the importance of setting limits and saying no to requests for more candy or the car keys, it may feel odd initially when they have to apply this to their eating-disordered teen's portion sizes ("I understand you feel full, but you need to finish"), physical complaints ("I'm sorry you don't feel well, but that's not a reason to skip lunch"), need for meal supervision ("I know none of your friends have their mom meet them at school for lunch, but that's something I need to do right now"), or apparent desires to be "healthy" ("I know you feel less anxious after a run, but at the moment, it's too dangerous for your body").

All of this is "for now," another core concept in FBT. Guiding your child back to their developmental path and putting food back in its place as a *part* of their lives—but not so central—is absolutely the goal. The duration of how long this can take varies. Some clients get better quickly, some need more time, and some relapse along the way. FBT is typically done over six to twelve months, and in three distinct phases that will be explained in greater detail in the following pages. In short, the phases start with understanding the illness and your new role in refeeding your child while implementing the Plate-by-Plate approach. Your child progresses to the second phase once they've achieved some success at weight and health restoration, and you'll welcome the third phase with your child regaining some or all food autonomy. This is much more a marathon than a sprint, and it is important to be prepared for the long haul while knowing it won't last forever.

Regardless of your particular path, both FBT and the Plate-by-Plate approach allow for adjustments as you go, with clear and manageable steps during what can seem like an unmanageable situation.

What Is FBT?

Throughout this book, our goal is for you to feel supported and coached on how to put meals and snacks together, in order to confidently help your child through nutritional rehabilitation, from beginning to end. These are primary goals of FBT, and the Plate-by-Plate approach has the advantage of being consistent with and supporting its principles.

Family-based treatment or FBT is considered as a treatment of approximately ten to twenty sessions carried out over the course of six to twelve months.[1] It is also known as the Maudsley approach, named after Maudsley Hospital in London where this particular type of treatment for eating disorders first originated in the 1980s. Specific to FBT are its three distinct treatment phases, as well as a number of key concepts. The table on page 34 summarizes FBT's treatment phases and key concepts, as well as how the Plate-by-Plate approach adds to treatment, which will be further outlined in the following pages.

The goal of FBT, as with recovery, is to effectively and efficiently establish weight restoration and health of the adolescent by viewing you, the parents, as the best resource to feed your child until they are able to resume appropriate eating on their own. FBT is considered a team approach, with parents being central to a multidisciplinary team of professionals, all working together on behalf of the adolescent suffering from an eating disorder.

Does FBT Really Work?

Yes! FBT has been shown to be highly effective. At the conclusion of treatment, 80 percent of patients are weight restored with the resumption of their menstrual cycle for girls, and 50 percent are fully remitted.[2] In fact, approximately two-thirds of adolescents with anorexia nervosa are recovered at the end of FBT, while 75 to 90 percent are fully weight recovered at a five-year follow-up.[3] With bulimia nervosa, FBT was found to be more effective in promoting abstinence from binge eating and purging than other therapies, such as cognitive behavioral therapy, at the end of treatment and the six-month follow-up.[4]

FBT is so highly regarded that most professionals in the field agree that all adolescents with anorexia nervosa should be offered a trial of FBT before any other treatment is considered. According to Dr. Daniel Le Grange, coauthor of *My Kid Is Back*, "Almost all studies involving adolescents with anorexia nervosa suggest that FBT is an effective therapy."[5] While Amanda Smith and Catherine Cook-Cottone note some challenges to this, they conclude that "in practice, those working with patients with AN should target family therapy as a first course treatment. Families have found aspects including refeeding to be helpful and research suggests that improvement of patient status is likely . . . Patients who show early signs of improvement have a greater likelihood to fare better."[6]

Early weight gain has been linked to the successful treatment of AN.[7] Achieving approximately a 3 percent weight gain by the fourth treatment session is a strong predictor of full remission; this translates to about four pounds of weight gain in the first four weeks. James Lock and other researchers reported that weight gain at sessions two and nine of FBT were both predictors of remission at twelve months.[8] In addition to weight gain, studies have identified other aspects—such as client age, duration of illness, other diagnoses including depression, anxiety and OCD, and parental conflict or challenges—that may signal the expectation for a longer treatment course or the need for additional treatment elements, such as parent coaching.[9]

Finally, if FBT is not an option, adolescent-focused therapy (AFT; a type of therapy done one-on-one between your child and a therapist), has been found to be a promising alternative. AFT is an individual psychotherapy approach that still focuses on the importance of weight gain and health but includes, from the outset, issues of adolescent self-discovery, autonomy, individuation, and assertiveness. A randomized clinical trial comparing

FBT with AFT for adolescents with anorexia nervosa was conducted by Lock et al, which found "that FBT is superior to AFT for adolescents with anorexia nervosa, though AFT remains an important alternative treatment for families that would prefer a largely individual treatment."[10] Again, the Plate-by-Plate approach has the advantage of being one you can use with all treatment variations described here.

Family-Based Treatment and the Plate-by-Plate Approach

PHASES	TYPICAL TIME FRAME	GOALS	KEY CONCEPTS	WHAT THE PLATE-BY-PLATE APPROACH ADDS
PHASE 1	Approximately ten weeks (Though in practice can take much longer)	Weight and health restoration, with parents in charge of refeeding Parents are able to take over all aspects/supervision of food and eating for now May include activity restrictions No focus on cause of the eating disorder or on other adolescent issues that do not pertain to weight and health restoration The family meal (usually second session) to explore what's working and what's challenging Looking for early weight gain as predictor of positive outcome; four pounds in four weeks Looking to avoid need for hospitalization or higher levels of care	Fighting *for* your teen and *against* the eating disorder, lovingly Helping your teen *get* better versus *feel* better Eating disorder is seen as external to your teen who has the illness Food as medicine Non-blame approach, as with most illnesses Parents are hands-on and united Helping parents find their confidence but no direction on specifics of meals Things can get worse before they get better	Agrees with all goals and concepts—weight-gain focus, non-blame, illness as external, parents as agents of change Introduce after family meal session Offers clarity of "dosing" the food as "medicine" Increases parent confidence Offers clarity and flexibility, while the eating disorder strives for rigidity and confusion Offers quick visual accuracy Easy to learn and to apply, in varied situations, and encourages parent alignment

PHASES	TYPICAL TIME FRAME	GOALS	KEY CONCEPTS	WHAT THE PLATE-BY-PLATE APPROACH ADDS
PHASE 2	Approximately seven weeks (Though, again, can take longer in practice)	Weight gain and compliance with parental oversight has been mostly accomplished Focus still on weight and health restoration with inclusion of other family issues *only* as they relate to weight, eating, and health. Weight gain continues (or stabilizes) while teen slowly begins to practice some food choice Gradual return to activity, as appropriate	Same concepts apply regarding no blame, illness as external, parents primarily in charge of the food, gradual reintroduction of teen autonomy with snacks and later with meals Parents tend to feel more confident and teen tends to be compliant Food is still medicine while gradually becoming less of the focus Avoid the temptation to rush this phase	Agrees with all concepts and helps with implementation of how and when to increase food autonomy Offers all the same ease of use, clarity of dosing and flexibility of previous phase Helps in the return to "normal" relationship with food
PHASE 3	Approximately three weeks	Teen can independently maintain weight above 95 percent of ideal weight and refrain from restriction in a variety of social settings Opportunity to explore issues that have necessarily been on hold, such as appropriate parental boundaries, issues of adolescence and autonomy, reestablishment of parental focus outside the eating disorder	"I've got my kid back!" Shift to *supporting* your child versus *fighting* the eating disorder Parents and teen are more collaborative Food resumes its proper place	Allows for small shifts to adjust for this big step, using all the same concepts Plates become part of eating intuitively, and not just a tool for refeeding

Phase 1: Refeeding Your Child and Achieving a Balanced Plate, AKA "All Hands on Deck"

The first phase of FBT is focused completely on addressing the eating disorder, where parents are "hands on" and oversee all aspects of their child's eating. The goals are weight and health restoration. At this stage you are actively fighting *for* your child and *against* the eating disorder. You completely manage the food; this means taking care of the grocery shopping, meal preparation, and plating, as well as total supervision of your child's eating. It will feel like an unusual task to take on with your adolescent who has been making many of their own food choices for the past several years, and flies in the face of their budding independence. It's like having one foot on the gas (helping them go into their life) and one foot on the brake (stopping their starvation). Like much of adolescence, it is doing a bit of both, but most parents never anticipate having to do this with food. This is where parents are both stretching themselves and also feeling diminished. With time and progress, you will become empowered and encouraged. Success will help motivate you to continue to fight against this all-encompassing disease.

This phase introduces many of the key concepts of FBT:

- Recognizing that the eating disorder is a serious illness that requires treatment
- Taking a non-blame or agnostic approach
- Externalizing the illness, where the child and the eating disorder are considered separate (i.e., "That's the eating disorder talking")
- Supporting parents to help them find their confident role in their child's recovery, building on their own wisdom, strength and love

On its own, however, FBT does not formally offer a specific method for refeeding your child, which is where the Plate-by-Plate approach (see page 101) comes in as an important supplement to FBT.

Finally, success in this first phase necessitates that parents agree with the goals of FBT, as well as participate in therapy sessions. (For more information about how to assemble your team of health professionals to aid you in this journey, see Chapter 3: It Takes a Village.) In this phase, the treatment team seeks to help parents manage a life-threatening illness that no one caused or wanted and that has become center stage in the family—"for now." Understanding that your child has an illness they didn't pick and cannot manage without intense intervention is paramount.

The nature of this illness, and in part why it is so lethal, is that your child will resist all attempts at treatment and a cure. It is not that dissimilar to a child requiring chemotherapy or surgery and absolutely not wanting to do those treatments out of fear and an understandable desire to avoid discomfort. In that situation, you would empathize with the fear but would not give in to it, and you would not allow the lifesaving treatment to be avoided or considered "optional." You would reassure your child that the treatment is necessary and that you will be there for your child, while also making them as comfortable as possible during the process. While your heart would go out to your child, your commitment to saving their life would not falter.

Eating disorders have the highest mortality rate of any psychiatric illness. While the illness tends to masquerade as a choice to be "healthy," once your child has the diagnosis, you must shift to recognizing that you are now facing a life-threatening illness.

As part of the blame-free approach, any questions of who or what caused the eating disorder are not judged or addressed. Whether or not families ate balanced meals together before the onset of the eating disorder is also not an area of right or wrong. Issues of past family positions on things like sugar consumption or attitudes toward fats are redirected in the now-known context of an eating disorder. If you see your child struggling in deep water, you don't spend time on whose fault it is that they are in the deep end or yell at them for not being a better swimmer. You just jump in and rescue them, even if they fight your efforts out of fear or confusion, and even if you've never been trained as a lifeguard. This is about saving your child, with love, concern, courage, and on-hand skill. The focus at this phase needs to be on getting your child nourished and their weight restored, not on how the eating disorder developed.

Confidently taking charge, plate by plate

Many parents feel overwhelmed as they begin to take such an active role in their child's recovery. Even though you've fed your child for their entire life, you may feel immobilized in the face of your child's eating disorder. Figuring out how to refeed a now eating-disordered child can be daunting. By the time an eating disorder is diagnosed, casual conversations about "what's for dinner" have morphed into tension-filled endeavors that leave everyone confused and exhausted. Here, the beauty of using the Plate-by-Plate approach to refeed your child really shines. It offers simple guidelines for how much food should be on their plate, what kind, and how often they should be eating. Just as the eating disorder wants to make meals much more complicated, the Plate-by-Plate approach "keeps it simple." So where the FBT approach offers parents a general map, the Plate-by-Plate approach adds a compass, both integral tools to help navigate the tricky terrain that is eating-disorder recovery. The exact route taken, however, is still very much in the hands of parents.

Typically, using FBT, parents are asked to "feed your child what *you* think they need to restore their health." Parents are guided primarily by the acknowledgment, in front of the child, that they are the most competent agents of change, and the treatment team will support the parents' efforts to "win" against the eating disorder, with every bite. All of this is not to make things more difficult for the parents but to be true to one of FBT's primary goals: to empower parents to be in charge of their child's nutrition and not undermine their confidence with a perceived need to rely on an expert or a particular meal plan.

In their *Treatment Manual for Anorexia Nervosa*, second edition, James Lock and Daniel Le Grange write, "It is important that the therapist be able to support the parents' explorations and attempts at weight restoration rather than providing them with a prescribed menu, calorie recommendations, or other formulas for recovery."[11] However, just like not all families improve with FBT, not all parents find this approach sufficient. Some parents have been openly frustrated feeling completely out of their league in determining the nuts and bolts of refeeding their anorexic child. In a parent-authored book by Eva Musby, *Anorexia and Other Eating Disorders*, Musby echoes what we hear from many parents, specifically that "many parents complain that they have been given no guidance on what to feed their child."[12]

In keeping with the understanding of the eating disorder as a serious illness, a parent once said, "I can support my child getting the medicine they need, but I don't think a doctor would ever leave the dose up to me." The Plate-by-Plate approach offers the structure of the "dose" without falling into the specifics that an eating disorder pulls for or implying that parents are incapable. It is consistent with the dire message that this is a life-threatening illness that requires food as medicine, with full parental participation, and with guidelines on how to proceed. It is the addition of this food "model" to FBT treatment that has led families to say, "Now I feel I can do this." With many of whom I've worked, it has allowed families to stay the course with FBT and to not give up. In Musby's book, as well as in *Survive FBT* by Maria Ganci, both authors offer general guidelines to give your child "what they need for weight recovery, rather than what you think they'll accept" as well as guidelines for weight gain and calories/day, with food as "medicine."[13]

The Plate-by-Plate approach helps parents move away from the worry of "Am I doing this right?" to a confident stance of "I've got this." Parents are definitely the ones in charge of refeeding, and the more comfortable you are with the Plate-by-Plate approach, the more confident you become. Even though it provides a model for your child's meals, it leaves a lot of room for your own judgment and wisdom. Does the meal "look like" the Plate-by-Plate approach? Does it look like a meal that will help restore your child's health? Parents are ultimately making that call.

There is no measuring or weighing food required, allowing you to take a stand against the eating disorder's desire to create doubt and to negotiate with you. Statements like "You gave me more rice than Mom did," "I don't need that much fat," or "I'm too full to eat any more," are common. FBT advises parents to hear your child's protests as "the eating disorder talking" (externalization of the illness as something separate from your child), and encourages them to stay the course of weight restoration and nutritional rehabilitation and not engage in eating disorder "negotiations."

Using the Plate-by-Plate approach, parents have reported having the structure to feel secure in the face of the eating disorder's arguments. It directly addresses the eating disorder's goal to create doubt and dilute the meal plan—all you need to do is take a fairly quick glance at the plate. The visual is a great advantage in the fight against an eating disorder, particularly as eating disorders are an exercise in both obfuscation and precise rigidity and detail. A parent once said, "It's like I can better ignore what the eating disorder is yelling at me, and I can just tune in to the plate and see what I've given is right. I can also see quickly if something is missing (if the eating-disordered child has thrown something out or given it to the dog)."

Another mother said, after her son completed treatment, "I came here exhausted, ready to give up, with no confidence at all in how to change things, and you gave me that. I know I can not only feed him (with the Plate-by-Plate approach) but challenge him the right way. I know what I'm doing."

All caregivers on the same page

The success of FBT depends on the degree to which parents are in agreement with the treatment and able to work together to deliver the "food as medicine," starting in this first phase. That parent alignment is associated with better outcomes makes sense, as the eating disorder will try to capitalize on any doubt or dissension, however small, between parents. Parental consistency has also been shown to be an important factor in terms of a child's weight gain.[14] In the FBT treatment manual, the authors note "the parents' success in refeeding their daughter can often directly be attributed to their ability to work as a team in this process," and that "parents need to be on the same line, the same page, the same word, at all times."[15] Parents ideally should be aligned as to the best treatment approach for their child, and should be in agreement about participating in FBT in order for the treatment to be successful.[16]

In her book *Survive FBT*, Ganci devotes a whole chapter to parent unity. Ganci writes, "Parents need to realize that refeeding an anorexic adolescent IS NOT normal parenting," about which parents can indeed offer differing opinions. "It is a prescription to get your child healthy and weight restored, therefore as a prescription, it needs to be administered in exactly the same way by both parents." The Plate-by-Plate approach helps parents and caregivers work together against the eating disorder, in that it is designed to make communication of "what" and "how much" the child needs to eat easier for all adults who are involved (parents, grandparents, caregivers, etc).

Everyone needs to agree that the goal of weight restoration is firm. Knowing simply what the plate should look like helps immensely with this. At times, the eating disorder will try to get parents to doubt themselves and back off. Plate-by-Plate instead offers a clear blueprint of what a meal or snack should look like that can be successfully implemented anywhere, and by any caregiver who understands it. Neither the eating disorder's drive for precision or chaos will interfere. It doesn't require exactness, and it also doesn't leave room for doubt. It's a model that encompasses parental strength and confidence, ease of use, flexibility of implementation, and simplicity.

The family meal session

Family-based treatment includes a family meal session. The family meal session, typically the second appointment in FBT, involves your therapist telling you to "bring a meal you think will help your child get better and gain weight" and should be completed before implementing the Plate-by-Plate approach. This session seeks to better understand the severity of your child's illness. It appreciates each family member's perspectives and strengths and begins to offer suggestions on how to be successful in refeeding your child. It is no more about judgment than a physician listening to your heart or reviewing a scan in order to evaluate how far the illness has encroached and how best to deliver the treatment and dose.

It can be an intense session and leave some parents feeling inadequate and protective of their child being asked to do something uncomfortable. But stick with it! The family meal session will help your therapist best understand how to guide you and also set the tone that you, the parents, are not backing down and will persevere over your child's eating disorder.

Expect pushback

The initial sessions of Phase 1 treatment are often very difficult for all family members. Your child will likely be angry and fearful about "losing control" over their diet and weight-loss goals. They will resist, even fight, your efforts to intervene. Prior to treatment, your child was providing excuses for avoiding eating, like "I'm not hungry" or "I already ate" or "I'm vegan now and can't eat that," and simply declined any efforts you may have made to get them to eat or take a day off from exercise. While you remained concerned, your child was firmly, but fairly quietly, holding their position. Once the eating disorder is cornered and challenged, however, this dynamic tends to change. Your child suddenly can appear angry, combative, and quite unexpectedly forceful in their response to your efforts to help. This can involve yelling, hitting, running away, throwing food, refusing to see providers, as well as hiding food or lying about behaviors.

At first, you might fear you made things worse by seeking treatment (and your child might try to convince you of this), when in fact you are actually seeing the strength of your child's eating disorder that was under wraps when left unchallenged. This is what it means when an FBT professional says, "This is the eating disorder talking."

Later in treatment, teens will often reflect back on the initial sessions and share that they were very difficult but also offered them a huge relief.

Until then, they had been dealing with the eating disorder on their own, usually frightened of their inability to stop their behaviors and deeply ashamed of their outbursts toward their parents. But with unquestionable and consistent parental intervention, they know help has arrived (though they likely won't thank you for a long time). A respected researcher and clinician in this field, Dr. Kathleen Kara Fitzpatrick, clinical assistant professor at Stanford and certified FBT therapist and trainer, talks about this as "hugging the iceberg." What parents typically first see as the illness in their child is really just the tip of the iceberg. Until you see it up close you can't realize the depth and seriousness of the illness. That you couldn't see the whole iceberg is not anyone's fault.

One set of parents who struggled in Phase 1 felt relief in recalling how growing up, their own parents enforced an unwavering curfew. They remembered how much they hated it, how they called their parents mean, how loud they argued and stomped around, how much they tried to negotiate. Underneath, however, they felt (a) cared for, (b) "off the hook" for having to leave the party early versus choosing to, and (c) relieved to not have to figure out these limits on their own. If curfew is ignored, there is a consequence; the child loses the privilege to go out with their friends for the next two weeks. This is exactly how it is with eating-disorder treatment. You, the parents, will hold the line, on behalf of your child's safety and well-being.

All of this is centered on a loving parental stance that can feel weird because it's about food, not misbehavior or drugs or alcohol. One individual recovering from anorexia shared "unlike addiction to cigarettes, drugs, and alcohol, in this type of rehab you can't abstain from the one thing that is causing the issue—food, you have to eat it." However, it's the same stance and consequences for not eating or for hiding food. There should be "natural consequences," such as needing to have a supplement at the next meal, or having the expectation that backpacks will be searched, or slumber parties disallowed. It is not about "punishment"; it is an appropriate response for a child with an illness. And it's one that lets your child clearly know that treatment is mandatory, not optional.

One parent said, "If my child gets mad at me about a meal, I know I'm fighting the eating disorder." And, of course, it is *not* the goal to upset your child, but it's a natural consequence of challenging the eating disorder. When your child engages in eating-disorder behaviors, they are not doing so willfully, rather they are being held hostage by the illness. It's a double-edged sword: your child cannot be freed without your help, and yet initially they will be unwilling participants in their own rescue.

Phase 2: Introducing Some Independence

The second phase begins only after the child shows compliance to parental refeeding and has made appropriate weight gain. In this phase, the pushback your child's eating disorder showed in Phase 1 will be much quieter. You will begin to feel increasingly confident about following the Plate-by-Plate approach, in various settings (whether a new restaurant or Thanksgiving at a grandparent's house). While weight is still discussed, it is with a greater sense of calm and optimism about the direction things are going.

This phase also marks the beginnings of gradually handing back some food participation to your child, for example, having your child pick their evening snack with your approval. You may ask your child to plate a meal on their own, with you standing by to make corrections if necessary. This gives your child the ability to reconnect with plating food, reminding them that one day they will do this completely on their own. They may begin to be allowed to eat out with friends, and therefore, without your supervision. Of course, combined with medical check-ins, you will receive feedback immediately as to whether some of the unsupervised meals are going okay. Keep in mind, your child has been looking at the plate you've been providing since treatment began and has by now learned what it should look like.

The Plate-by-Plate approach is inexact by design, which helps jumpstart a more "normal" food dialogue in Phase 2. Helping your child put together a snack no longer involves an eating-disorder-driven conversation about calories or fat grams but merely what a snack should "look like." It is important not to underestimate what a relief this will be to your teen. Most adolescents recovering from an eating disorder do not want to *ever* think about calories or numbers again, and it is in the best interest of their recovery that they don't.

Phase 2 is meant to be a gradual shift, and it is still necessary to oversee your child's eating throughout this phase. You will continue to be involved, and that can be hard for those parents who arrive at Phase 2 completely exhausted, eager to put this illness behind them, and ready to hand back all autonomy to their teen. This is similar to being at the halfway mark of a marathon, and you will need to pace yourself to make it to the finish line. Just like when your child began to learn to walk, you didn't immediately disappear but stayed nearby to catch them when they fell as they practiced this new skill. For your child, venturing back into the realm of food choices, without the eating disorder, is like a whole new stage of development. Your child will not simply go back to life before the eating disorder, though life will feel more normal. Fears of certain foods, exercise compulsions, and worry about weight are still going on in your child's mind, although they are quieter. If you think about healing from a broken leg, this phase is tantamount to the cast coming off but still needing physical therapy, using a boot and crutches, and knowing your leg doesn't look normal yet. And for some, even a broken leg might mean changing forever the sports you engage in, or being more cautious, or expecting future surgeries. Eating-disorder recovery can be very much the same.

While the transition to Phase 2 can go quite smoothly, for some teens, entering Phase 2 may quickly allow the eating disorder to come roaring back in. With more food autonomy, your child might skip a snack here and there, or there might be an increase in their food negotiations and pushback. One parent discovered food hidden again in shoes and drawers. Trust your instincts. If it looks like the eating disorder is back, then act like it's back until you know otherwise. Teens often pull out the "You don't trust me!" complaint, and the answer is: "I don't trust the eating disorder, and if I can't tell if it's the eating disorder or not,

I'm going to assume it is until I know for sure." Adding back more supervision and pulling back on autonomy might be indicated if your child begins to struggle more in this phase.

Recovery from an eating disorder really requires clear evidence of improvement before backing off, not just the hope of improvement. In other areas of parenting, hoping for improvement makes complete sense. Parents may stop nagging about homework in hope that their teen will start to set their own study habits and learn to be more accountable. But with eating disorders, "hope" frequently gets co-opted by the eating disorder and used as an opportunity to return. If the eating disorder sneaks back in, this is not a failure but simply what can happen with illness. (Again, it is no one's fault.)

When this happens, the usual wisdom is "go back to the last time it worked" until compliance and weight gain are back to where you think a Phase 2 attempt can be tried again. You may resume some, not necessarily all, of your successful Phase 1 activities, like adding caloric beverages with all meals, or supervised school lunches, or delay of participation in a school sport until you and your child are ready to try increasing their autonomy again.

Phase 3: Helping Your Child Get Back to Normal

The third and final phase is the one in which you, the parents, get to shift from *actively fighting* the eating disorder to *supporting* your child. It typically feels different, like you are back to being on the same team, recovering together from something that everyone has gone through. This phase begins when the adolescent is able to independently maintain weight above 95 percent of median BMI and refrains from food restriction in a variety of social settings. This is where you and your child come back together in a more collaborative approach and allow for discussion of not only food and eating but also other issues that have necessarily been on hold during the time of illness and treatment.

In Phase 3, parents begin to say, "I've got my kid back!" Your child is no longer starving and is weight restored, yet they may still have body-image concerns or fears about certain foods or numbers. Some families have been so traumatized by the impact of the illness that shifting to this phase feels as scary as starting treatment. Parents, who have been told they have a central role in recovery, understandably struggle to now relinquish this huge responsibility. And, it is often the case that some eating disorder debris will periodically wash up. This might happen when your child is invited to a swim party and begins to worry about their body shape, or when they go to college and quickly lose weight, or they resume their sport and they simply can't keep up with their increased metabolic needs. Again, as in Phase 2, trust your instincts. You now have the advantage of knowing what the eating disorder looks like, which you didn't know at the beginning. You'll see it, if it returns, and you'll know what to do.

This is why the Plate-by-Plate approach serves you so well. By Phase 3, you are not changing to a whole new meal plan or new way of thinking about meals, but simply tweaking the plate for this stage of recovery. For example, knowing how to put a plate together at any dining hall has been immensely helpful to families sending recovered teens to college.

The benefits of the Plate-by-Plate approach cannot be overstated by the time you reach this stage. Families attempting to make treatment transitions using more rigid methods like tracking exchanges or calories have struggled to understand and implement these plans. Teens have also become stuck in the particulars of following such a plan. Exchanges become an exacting "specific way to eat" that reinforces all that the eating disorder holds dear—that there is only *one* way to eat, that you have to be *very* careful, that precision is necessary for our health and weight, and that uncalculated food cannot be tolerated or eaten. And it also reinforces peculiar eating behaviors that we want the teens to move away from. Most providers who use exchanges or calories in their treatment completely acknowledge their use was meant as temporary. But even temporary use creates an additional step in recovery ("getting off exchanges" or "discontinuing food measurements") that wouldn't be necessary if they were never introduced in the first place.

The Plate-by-Plate approach deftly sidesteps this dilemma by creating a plan that transitions seamlessly as your child recovers.

By Phase 3, most pushback—the eating disorder's "arguments" about the Plate-by-Plate approach—has diminished, making this phase, appropriately, not about food at all but about getting back into life without an eating disorder. Plate-by-Plate becomes a tool for finding balance and variety at all meals throughout one's life.

Finally: You've Got This!

In a recent movie about a teenager recovering from anorexia, one parent comments to another that trying family-based treatment was "brave." In the movie, they seem to imply that FBT is only for the heroic few who attempt it. But that underestimates the power of an approach founded on a parent's instinct to protect their child. There are other avenues one can take to help your child recover, although none are as successful with teens as FBT and offer the support of having a team alongside you. It is certainly not an easy path, but most illnesses and their treatments share the necessity of hard work, perseverance, and patience.

FBT is meant to be a loving and effective tool, which empowers parents to get their child not only back but also back into their regular adolescent lives. It is *not* about "forcing your child to eat" but about ensuring your child adheres to the lifesaving treatment, with love, support, and reassurance. Parents often express doubt, confusion, and even resistance when first learning what is required to help their child recover from an eating disorder. However, they also report upon successful completion of treatment that FBT, together with the Plate-by-Plate approach, gave them the tools they needed to not only start the treatment but also see it through. Getting your child back from an eating disorder is a search and rescue mission like nothing you've ever done, and having a child reappear from their eating disorder is something you'll never forget. In the spirit of FBT: you've got this!

CHAPTER 3

———

It Takes a Village

Getting Help from Your Team

*"Why does my child have so many appointments?
I can't take this much time off work!"*

*"We haven't told our friends and family what's going on with
our child because we're worried they won't understand."*

"I'm completely exhausted; I need a vacation!"

Getting Help from Your Inner Circle

IF YOUR CHILD had cancer, would you tell your family and friends? How about if they got in a terrible car accident and needed to be hospitalized? It is likely that you would seek solace from your community for love, prayers, and support.

Likewise, those who are struggling with eating disorders need huge amounts of support—and so do the families who care for them. Individuals with eating disorders have significantly elevated mortality rates, with the highest rates occurring in those with anorexia nervosa.[1] Unfortunately, mental illness is often stigmatized in our society and can cause parents to feel immense shame and guilt. While it may seem hard to open up to your community about your struggles, it will be much harder to enter this battle alone. Now is the time to trust your closest family members and friends, to educate them about the severity of eating disorders and the amount of work and dedication it takes from the entire family to successfully manage and treat it. Although not everyone may understand what you are going through, you will discover through this process who you can trust and rely on in the hardest of times.

As discussed in chapter 2, family-based treatment—where parents take charge of their child's recovery—is a highly effective treatment option for adolescents with eating disorders. However, without enough support, parents and other caregivers often burn out from the process. It can be a grueling, exhausting, long, and bumpy road. Caring for your teen may feel as if you have a toddler again, one who has frequent tearful tantrums in response to not getting what they want. And the pressure to succeed couldn't be higher; your child's life, health, and happiness depend on successful intervention. You may find you feel constantly worried about your child's health, in addition to the worries that you already had such as whether they are safe, happy, finishing their homework, and going to bed on time. Undoubtedly, you may even question whether what you are doing is helpful and whether there is "something more" you could be doing. When you have enough support you are better able to tap into your own parental instinct, which will guide you through this process.

Because the process of taking back control of the dinner table can look strange to those who aren't familiar with eating disorders, you will need to educate your support group so they can lift you up when you need it most. Otherwise, your family and friends may question everything you are tasked with to care for your child and they may end up saying something more hurtful than helpful. They will wonder why your sixteen-year-old needs you to eat lunch with them at school every day or why your fourteen-year-old isn't allowed to make an after-school snack on their own. They won't understand why you can't bring the family over for a barbecue or will feel hurt when you cancel, again, on the plans you made to go out to a movie. Your support group needs to understand why you cannot leave your child alone and why all meals must be closely supervised. Share with them that the nature of eating disorders is highly secretive, and at this early stage of treatment, you can't trust your child right now to tell you the truth about food or exercise.

It is also incredibly common for family members to talk about weight or diets in front of a child with an eating disorder without even realizing that what they are saying fuels the disorder. Please refer to Chapter 12: How to Talk About Diet and Weight (Hint: Don't!) for further information about this sensitive topic.

When your friends and family have a background on what you are facing every day, they can be more effective in supporting you through this process. Some families, recognizing and appreciating the new-found support, have even had their friends and family join in some of the medical and therapy sessions to learn more, or to join them for a support group meeting.

Including your inner circle in meals can be helpful to give you a break while giving your child the opportunity to hear the same message from yet another person. It will take a little work up front from you to teach your inner circle how to supervise meals, be supportive of your child, and to hold the line during mealtime crises. This is no different than if you needed a family member to provide medicine for your child while you are away, or a trusted babysitter to learn how to manage your toddler's mealtime tantrums. If you teach them and allow them to fumble while they practice, they will help support you, making the long-term outcome more successful.

Getting Help from Professionals

In order for FBT and the Plate-by-Plate approach to be most effective, we recommend that you hire a strong multidisciplinary team specialized in the treatment of adolescent eating disorders. The team consists of:

- A **medical provider**, to monitor your child's weight, vital signs, hormones, and lab work
- A **family-based therapist**, to work closely with your child and your family

- A **registered dietitian**, to guide the Plate-by-Plate approach
- Possibly a **psychiatrist**, if recommended, to assess if medications may be helpful

This team is your extra set of hands in treating your child's eating disorder and you will build a strong relationship with them. You should trust them to help you and your child along through this process, and trust that they have your family's best interest in mind. The team will communicate often, and each member will share updates from the last appointment with the other providers in order to create a helpful plan of action. They should be consistent in their messages to you and your child so that there is no room for your child's eating disorder to "split" the team or negotiate about treatment recommendations. This will help you feel empowered and help you be consistent with your messages at home. To move things along, typically families will want to meet with these providers weekly, with these appointments continuing for as long as necessary to get your child to a safe, weight-restored place.

This team of specialists will help you learn how to effectively treat your child with an eating disorder. Here is a summary of each clinician's role in helping your child to recover:

Medical provider

At this point, you may have already paid a visit to the pediatrician concerning your child's declining weight and vital signs. Unless that pediatrician is comfortable managing the complex medical needs of a child with an eating disorder, they will refer you and your child to a medical provider who specializes in the treatment of eating disorders. There are many highly complex medical complications that arise as a result of malnutrition, and these must be addressed quickly and be closely monitored to provide the greatest chance of a full recovery. Please refer to chapter 4 for a detailed account of what to expect from your child's medical provider.

Therapist

As discussed in chapter 2, your child will benefit greatly from strong family-based treatment with a trained FBT-certified therapist. The therapist will require weekly sessions, at a minimum, and will ask that both parents attend each session. The family-based therapist will guide you in how to take back your dinner table, while coaching you to develop strong FBT skills.

Registered dietitian

Ideally, your child will work with a registered dietitian (RD) during this process. Just like physicians, not all dietitians specialize in the treatment of eating disorders. The RD you hire for you and your child will need a strong understanding of eating disorders as well as family-based treatment and should work closely with the rest of the multidisciplinary team. A solid understanding of the Plate-by-Plate approach will help to make treatment seamless and prevent treatment confusion.

The initial RD visit will be mostly about gathering information—speaking with you and your child both separately and together about what has been going on at home. Eating disorders are secretive, and an individual struggling with an eating disorder is more likely to open up to the RD when their parents are not present. In the same fashion, you will want to speak with the RD alone in order to discuss openly any struggles you have been dealing with in trying to feed and care for your child during this difficult time. While most of this initial session will include questions that are historical in nature, the RD will also begin educating you about the Plate-by-Plate approach and how to proceed at home. Toward the end of the appointment they will also provide guidance to you and your child together about the initial stages of this treatment approach. You will be expected to attend weekly follow-up visits, with discussion about how meals have been going and what your child is eating. The RD will then help create a plan for how to build on the previous week's progress.

Psychiatrist

Your child may also be referred to a psychiatrist who will perform an initial assessment and determine whether your child may benefit from psychiatric medications. While medications do not cure eating disorders, there are some medications that help manage symptoms of eating disorders and other psychological concerns such as anxiety, depression, or obsessive-compulsive disorder (OCD) (should the psychiatrist find any of them to be present in your child). Your child may have underlying anxiety or depression, for example, and medications can be helpful.

Every recommendation will be made by your treatment team in order to help your child recover as quickly as possible. Some recommendations may be hard to hear, and difficult to implement, but an experienced team usually makes those recommendations for a reason. At the same time, your input on these decisions is important—sometimes what seems reasonable to providers might be totally off to you as the parent. You may not understand why your child's RD is asking you to increase your child's plates further, or why your therapist is recommending that you bring in your other children to session. You may disagree with the psychiatrist's recommendation to start an antidepressant, or the physician's recommendation to stop all activity. Good communication is of utmost importance during treatment and it is imperative that everyone is on the same page. Feel free to speak up and express your concerns to the team. You may wish to receive more information from your team to better understand their recommendations. Your treatment team should be able to provide you with sound, evidence-based explanations.

Your child may become upset during an appointment when they hear something they don't like: "You need to gain more weight," or "You can't exercise," or "You need to eat more," or "You can't go to the sleepover," or "You have to stay home from camp." Remember, these recommendations, though difficult and disappointing, are made in the interest of helping your child recover from an eating disorder. Stay focused on what's best for your child, and don't let the meltdown sway that conviction. And no doubt, your child will need extra love and support during these difficult times.

A child suffering from an eating disorder typically becomes a master negotiator, looking for any holes and cracks to exploit. If your child is upset because the physician will not authorize activity this week for example, try to present a unified front with the provider as much as possible. This allows there to be no wiggle room. You can remind your child that physical rest is required for the body to protect itself and to heal. Provide support to your child by letting them know that you will help them find other ways to fill their time. Suggest to your child that you can swing by the library to get new books, or create a space for art in the house and fill it with art supplies. Consider visiting an animal shelter or seeing a movie one afternoon.

Know that your child may become so distraught in the face of a provider's recommendations that there is almost nothing in the moment that you can do, other than hold them (if they will let you) and sit with them, until the intensity of the emotion dissipates. It is also equally likely that your child may appear totally fine during an appointment but then unravel as soon as you get into the car. Allow your child to be upset and to grieve as long as they are not a danger to you, their self, or anyone else. If you and your child are safe, it is okay for your child to be angry. If they are inconsolable, suggest deep breathing, or let them know you hear them, love them, and care deeply about them. Acknowledge their discomfort and remind them that while this may seem to be the end of the world as they know it, it will not always be this way. Remind your child that their continued work toward recovery will help them gain their life back and that you are there to support them through the struggle.

If your child does become a danger to themselves or anyone in your family—for example, if they kick or hit you or anyone else out of anger, if they threaten to jump out of the car on the way home, if they even suggest they would rather die than to continue treatment—even if you don't think they are serious, you must show them how seriously you take their words and actions. Call 911 or head to the nearest emergency room for evaluation. It's better to be safe than sorry in these instances, and since eating disorders are a very serious mental illness, they should be regarded as such. Your local police department and emergency department are part of your village and are not there to judge you but to help you keep your child safe from the dangers of their eating disorder.

Taking Care of You

Feeding your child three meals and at least two snacks a day, every day, when each meal is a battle, can be overwhelming and, frankly, exhausting. You may be asking yourself, after weeks or months of treatment, whether this is sustainable. Some parents choose to take a leave of absence from their job during this time. Perhaps you did that and now that time is up. What do you do? How do you get the help you need so that you can continue to fight for your child?

The first step is to talk with your support system and treatment team about how you are feeling. Ask if your spouse or other adult family members can pitch in more in order to relieve you. Take stock of each other's skill sets and formulate a plan to divide and conquer in the face of your child's eating disorder. Are you the calmest caregiver at mealtimes, or do you become easily frustrated? Perhaps you could do meal prep and leave the mealtime supervision to your spouse. Can your spouse or parent take over dinner and evening snack when you are exhausted? Is there a grandparent who can move in with you for a while to help?

Are you exhausted from the constant cooking? Perhaps you need some relief in meal preparation. If so, you may want to look into meal delivery services or grocery delivery programs that use an app to deliver food right to your house (for example, Peapod, Instacart, Munchery, FreshDirect, Amazon Prime Pantry, AmazonFresh, or Google Express). This has the added benefit of adding variety to your child's diet. Quick and easy frozen meals might save time as well. You may consider asking if any family, friends, or neighbors can help in the responsibilities of grocery shopping and meal preparation.

Are you taking care of yourself? Do you get enough sleep at night? Similar to caring for a sick loved one, caregivers must take care of themselves in order to successfully help their loved one. During times of distress on an airplane, passengers are instructed to first put the oxygen mask on themselves, before they can assist someone else. Think about what it's like to care for a three-year-old who wears you down—you are much better equipped to manage the child when you are well-rested and well-fed. These days, your teen needs you to be rested enough to help them battle this eating disorder, and you cannot do this alone.

Consider getting your own individual therapist to talk to. In the darkest moments of eating-disorder treatment, you may find that you can't remember the last time you went out on a date, put on makeup or shaved, or put on dressy clothes. You may not be exercising anymore because of worry that it will send the wrong message to your child. Perhaps this was previously your favorite way to destress and unwind and now you've lost a major coping mechanism. At what felt like the abyss of eating-disorder treatment, one parent apologized in session: "I haven't even brushed my teeth today," and then burst into tears. This is not uncommon; you are being stretched to new limits, and this work is tough. Your child's recovery relies heavily on your well-being, and since this may be a long process, you will need to pace yourself in order to get through this tiring journey.

Your village is there to support you, to listen to you, to comfort you, your child, and the rest of your family as you face what is likely to be the most challenging time in your life. It starts with your recognizing what you need and not being afraid to ask for help. Do not be ashamed of your child's illness. The more you can share, the more support will funnel back toward you. If you are struggling to find support people, please refer to the resources on page 275 for more help.

CHAPTER 4

⚊⚊⚊🍴⚊⚊⚊

Common Medical Issues

By Susanne Martin, MD

⎯⎯⎯⎯⎯⎯⎯⎯⎯⎯⎯⎯⎯⎯⎯⎯⎯⎯⎯⎯⎯⎯⎯⎯

AS YOU OBSERVE your child getting thinner and thinner, you may find yourself becoming increasingly worried. "How can my child possibly be exercising *this much* while eating *so* little? Is their heart okay?" Or you might be alarmed to find out that your child has been vomiting after every meal they eat. You may wonder if your child has an eating disorder, or whether they have an entirely different underlying medical condition. You have a right to be concerned, as these behaviors can lead to medical complications that affect almost every system in the body. If you are worried that your child might be suffering from an eating disorder, or if they have drastically changed their diet and exercise routine, it's a good idea to schedule an appointment with your child's pediatrician. They will discuss your concerns and do a complete physical exam with blood work to assess your child's current medical status and rule out other causes for weight loss, malnutrition, or vomiting. This chapter will outline what medical complications you should be concerned about, and what to expect from your medical provider.

Body Systems Affected by Malnutrition

Cardiovascular

We've found that parents are often most worried about how their child's heart is affected by malnutrition. A careful assessment of your child's cardiac functioning can be done easily in the outpatient setting.

Malnutrition and weight loss cause a person's vital signs to become unstable (such as with low blood pressure, low pulse, changes from a lying to standing position, or cold body temperature). These are changes that represent abnormalities to the functioning of the heart:

- Decreased overall cardiac mass including thinning of the heart muscle
- Reduced chamber volume, which means that the heart chambers push less blood volume out with each beat
- Protrusion of heart valves may cause mitral valve prolapse, in which the valve between the upper and lower left chambers of the heart becomes floppier and may not close properly.
- Fibrosis, which is the excess accumulation of stiff fiber (called matrix) into the cardiac muscle
- Pericardial effusion, which is a fluid collection around the heart and can lead to increased pressure surrounding the heart (this can negatively affect the heart function)

Malnutrition causes vital-sign instability and is often one of the main reasons for medical hospitalization. Typical instabilities include: a low resting heart rate of fewer than fifty beats per minute (defined as bradycardia, see page 60), low blood pressure with a systolic reading (the numerator of a blood pressure reading) of fewer than ninety (hypotension), EKG abnormalities, and orthostasis (inability to adjust heart rate and blood pressure appropriately with a change in position from lying to standing), among others. Your child's heart rate is assessed simply by taking your child's pulse in the office after resting. The heart rate is then measured in different positions, lying to standing.

Orthostatic hypotension refers to a drop in systolic blood pressure from lying to standing of more than twenty millimeters mercury.

Orthostatic tachycardia refers to a heart rate change between lying and standing of more than twenty beats per minute.

Bradycardia is defined as a heart rate of fifty beats per minute or fewer, and is commonly seen in patients with eating disorders.

Medical hospitalization might be indicated with any of the aforementioned cardiovascular instabilities. Families may try to blame their child's low heart rate on their athleticism and may even report that they themselves have a low resting heart rate. However, in a growing child, this low heart rate can be dangerous and originates from a weakened heart due to poor nutrition, not a strong athletic heart. The main concern with a sustained low heart rate is the risk of arrhythmias (irregularities of the heartbeat) and sudden cardiac arrest. Of note, a heart rate reading is often lower at night, so if your child goes to the doctor and their heart rate is forty-five beats per minute during the day, it will be even lower in the middle of the night. This is why a child with a very low heart rate will often be hospitalized. In the hospital, doctors, nurses, and other medical staff will closely monitor and assess the heart as well as other vital signs, and provide an increase in nutrition and fluids as needed to correct malnutrition-related vital-sign instabilities. In extreme and somewhat rare cases of bradycardia requiring hospitalization, a bedside pacer or defibrillator and admission to the intensive care unit (ICU) may be warranted.

With increased caloric intake, bradycardia will improve, but often at a very slow rate. Weeks of hospitalization are not unusual for an improvement in bradycardia, which can be frustrating for parents who are eager to hear of improvements in vital signs. Orthostatic blood-pressure changes usually resolve within several days of initial nutritional rehabilitation, but orthostatic pulse changes usually take several weeks to resolve. Orthostatic changes might not require hospitalization and can be monitored closely in the outpatient level of care. We highly discourage you to monitor your child's vital signs on your own. This responsibility and interpretation should be left to your child's medical provider.

Blood Abnormalities

The most common electrolyte disturbances that occur in the context of an eating disorder include low serum potassium, sodium, phosphorus, and magnesium.

- **Low potassium, or hypokalemia,** is primarily a result of vomiting, or laxative and diuretic abuse
- **Low sodium, or hyponatremia,** often occurs from excessive water intake, a behavior sometimes used to falsify weight or suppress hunger. Excessive water consumption, known as "water intoxication" and sometimes seen in patients with eating disorders, can lead to seizures, coma, and even death. Both low sodium and low potassium can be corrected within twenty-four to forty-eight hours.
- **Low phosphorus, or hypophosphatemia,** is indicative of "refeeding syndrome," which refers to a dangerous constellation of medical complications often resulting from aggressive renourishment. Phosphorus is known to play an important role in cardiac and brain function. Phosphorus levels are usually in the normal range during malnutrition, but upon refeeding, can drop rapidly.[3] Phosphorus levels drop significantly in 27.5 percent of patients admitted to the hospital and typically reach their lowest level within the first week of refeeding.[4] A sudden drop in phosphorus can cause cardiac arrhythmias, and mental status changes including confusion, anxiety, and irritability.

    As your child begins the refeeding process, medical monitoring is necessary to ensure that phosphorus levels remain normal, or if they do drop, that a supplement is provided. In the inpatient setting, it is not uncommon to replace phosphorus orally or intravenously and to check electrolyte levels at least once daily.

- **Low magnesium, or hypomagnesemia,** can continue for months, requiring oral supplementation and regular monitoring to raise magnesium levels
- **Low glucose, or hypoglycemia,** is common during the refeeding process. This can result from a fasting glucose level and/or be seen after eating (known as "reactive hypoglycemia"). Recent studies indicate that individuals who are older have a higher risk of hypoglycemia.[5] Normal glucose levels range between 100–140 mg/dL (milligrams per deciliter) two hours after eating, yet during the refeeding process, it is not uncommon to observe glucose levels in the forties (mg/dL) without any symptoms. Some treatment centers include hypoglycemia as a criterion for medical hospitalization, as normalization of glucose levels can take several weeks in the outpatient level of care.

There are several other abnormalities that may show up in your child's blood work:

- **High liver transaminases (AST and ALT):** Liver transaminases are enzymes that are elevated in almost half of all patients with AN.[6] Weight loss and fasting can produce mild elevation (two to three times the normal) of transaminases. Mild transaminase elevation (also known as steatosis) can also occur early in the course of refeeding and can take weeks to months to resolve.
- **High amylase levels:** Amylase is an enzyme, primarily in saliva and pancreatic fluid, which converts starch and glycogen into simple sugars. High levels can be found with regular binging, purging, or vomiting.
- **Abnormal blood urea nitrogen (BUN) and creatinine markers:** BUN can be low or high, and creatinine markers (generally used to assess kidney function) are high. Abnormal numbers result from low muscle mass and dehydration. In this context, it is reversible and usually not life-threatening.
- **Abnormal hematology:** With starvation, the bone marrow's normal production of all cell lines (mainly white cells, red cells, and plate-

lets) can be impaired and markedly decreased. Anemia (a low red-cell count), leukopenia (low white-cell count), or thrombocytopenia (low platelet count) in a pattern involving one, two, or all three cell lines can occur simultaneously. To the untrained eye, this might look like an underlying hematologic problem but is fully reversible with improved nutrition. Further workup may be necessary, however, to rule out any other cause of illness.

- **Vitamin/mineral deficiencies:** Iron deficiency and vitamin deficiencies, including vitamin D, vitamin B12, and others often result from poor overall food intake in addition to strict vegetarianism or veganism without appropriate education and management. Blood work to check these levels may be recommended.

- **Elevated lipid panels** (the panel of blood tests that serve as a screening tool for abnormalities in lipids such as cholesterol and triglycerides): Ironically, we also see elevated lipid panels in malnourished patients with AN. You may think of elevated cholesterol, triglycerides, and other lipids as something that occurs primarily in overweight individuals due to genetics and poor diet, however, during malnutrition, total cholesterol, LDL (low density lipoprotein), and HDL (high density lipoprotein) can be elevated as well. Elevated levels of cholesterol increase the risk for heart attacks and other forms of cardiovascular disease later in life. There have been several theories regarding the pathophysiology of these cholesterol abnormalities and include reduced cholesterol metabolism, starvation-induced increase of cholesterol transport from the periphery to the liver, or decreased LDL-receptor activity. Our bodies, which can naturally produce cholesterol, may overproduce cholesterol in the absence of a diet that contains cholesterol (found in animal foods) and enough fat. In most of these cases, improved nutrition, and particularly the incorporation of fats and cholesterol, returns cholesterol levels to baseline (unless the high cholesterol levels predate the eating disorder). You may find it surprising to add more fats and cholesterol into your child's diet to lower cholesterol levels. We often hear, "I should add more fats to my child's diet, even though their cholesterol is so high?" Yes, during times of malnutrition when a restricted diet is evident, adding more fats and cholesterol will suppress the body's own cholesterol production thus reducing blood cholesterol levels back to a normal range.

Visible Changes

As a parent, you might have noticed physical changes in your child's body. You may see their bones protruding, or their eyes may appear to be sunken. You may see muscle wasting or cachexia; cheek fullness (this is generally more pronounced in adolescents who purge); dry or dull skin (which can crack and bleed, especially on the fingers and toes); fine hair growth on arms, cheeks, or back called lanugo (an attempt of the body to conserve heat); hair loss and thinner hair; and brittle nails.

Hair loss

Visible hair loss and hair thinning, as well as brittle nails, might not be noticeable until about three months after the peak of malnutrition. During malnutrition, the hair follicles go into a resting phase—there is simply not enough extra fuel around to stimulate normal hair growth and regeneration. Hair loss can sometimes increase during refeeding as the hair cycle wakes up and begins to produce new hair. This causes some of the hair that was stuck in the resting phase to fall out. This can be quite alarming for kids, especially as they are eating more, but it symbolizes that the body is getting back on track again. Hair loss might last weeks to months, but usually improves with time.

Skin

You may have also noticed that your child is always cold. This is known as "cold intolerance." Their hands and feet might feel cold, and they may be bundling up in many layers. Sweatshirts and sweaters of course make it hard to notice that your child has lost weight. During malnutrition, it is common to see a bluish discoloration of the tips of the fingers as well as the nose and ears (known as acrocyanosis). The body no longer has enough energy to maintain cardiovascular function to keep your child warm and is prioritizing to send blood to the most vital organs. Bruising and skin sores are due to poor stores of fat beneath the skin and are a common physical symptom of malnutrition.

Jaundice

Another symptom is a yellowish coloration of the skin (jaundice) caused by either hyperbilirubinemia (a buildup of a yellow pigment called bilirubin) or hypercarotenemia (a buildup of beta-carotene in the body. Hyperbilirubinemia reflects that the liver isn't working properly.

A less serious cause of jaundice (not limited to eating disorders) can be from consuming too much beta-cartene. Beta-carotene is a pigment found in many fruits and vegetables, such as carrots, dark leafy greens, winter squash, sweet potatoes, and cantaloupe. Normally, the body converts beta-carotene to vitamin A, eliminating the presence of any abnormal pigment in the skin. However, an excessive intake of beta-carotene can cause the skin to take on a yellow or orange hue. This is especially pronounced on the palms of the hands, soles of the feet, and, to a lesser degree, the face. As a child improves medically, they will become less orange over time.

Gastrointestinal (GI) Disturbances

Malnutrition, and then the process of refeeding, can cause gastrointestinal distress, including bloating, fullness, gas, and alterations in bowel function. A malnourished child may have additional gastrointestinal symptoms such as early satiety, nausea, vomiting, and heartburn. Often, anxiety, muscle tension, and poor posture during meals can contribute to the feeling of nausea. Here we have highlighted some other gastrointestinal concerns.

Delayed emptying from the stomach

Medically, this is known as "gastroparesis" which develops with food restriction and weight loss. Gastroparesis is common and causes kids to feel bloated and full, especially after eating. Usually, when someone eats, the food is digested in a direct path: the food goes into the mouth, then into the stomach, to the small intestine, to the large intestine, and then eventually out of the body in the form of stool (which by that point is just waste, as all the key nutrients have been absorbed). During malnutrition, this process is delayed, particularly as it leaves the stomach. It takes an improved diet, where the person is not only eating more but also eating frequently, to push the metabolism and digestion along. In our experience, it may take four to five days of being consistent with one's diet before the rate of digestion can improve, even if just slightly. From there, usually the amount one is eating is further increased, and the metabolism/rate of digestion continues to improve.

Reduced digestive enzymes

Malnutrition can cause a reduction in the production of lactase, the enzyme needed to digest milk, or lipase, the enzyme needed to digest fat.[7] A child with an eating disorder may experience a temporary lactose intolerance or have trouble digesting high-fat foods. This makes it more challenging to accomplish the task of refeeding. However, these difficulties in digestion are temporary and resolve with improved nutrition. With time, lactase and lipase levels increase back to normal.

Gastrointestinal disturbances

With increased meal volume and frequency, your child will most likely feel full and have some level of gastrointestinal discomfort. They may feel bloated and have an increase in gas production, which are both normal symptoms experienced while the body is undergoing the metabolic and physiologic changes associated with the refeeding process. There may be a reduction or an increase in bowel movements. It can be helpful to reassure your child that the bowel patterns in healthy adolescents vary anywhere from two to three times per day to three times per week, and that adolescents with extensive weight loss have even fewer bowel movements. Your child should know that there is nothing fundamentally wrong with their gastrointestinal system other than a need for weight gain through improved nutrition.

Superior mesenteric artery (SMA) syndrome

SMA is a rare but notable gastrointestinal complication in patients with AN and results from compression of the small intestine (duodenum). In cases of severe malnutrition, a loss of the fat pad that normally surrounds the SMA compresses the duodenum between the aorta and spine posteriorly and the SMA anteriorly. This is a direct result of rapid weight loss. SMA syndrome manifests with severe upper-quadrant abdominal pain soon after eating, along with early satiety, nausea, and vomiting. The pain associated with SMA is debilitating, and vomiting might be intractable. An abdominal CT scan or an upper GI series are primarily used for diagnosis of this rare syndrome, and feedings through a specialized nasal tube into the intestines during hospitalization is necessary.

Our philosophy is to let the food heal the body naturally and to use pharmaceuticals only on a limited basis. You and your child's treatment team should acknowledge the discomfort and show an understanding without giving the eating disorder an excuse to "eat less." Supportive measures include heating pads, breathing and relaxation exercises, stretching, distraction, and other tools that can be taught by the therapist. Rarely, medications may be prescribed—such as ondansetron (Zofran) for nausea and/or metoclopramide (Reglan, though used less often)—that stimulate stomach contraction and hasten emptying of the stomach.

Hormonal Changes

During an initial medical assessment, blood levels of hormones should be evaluated. Malnutrition results in low levels of the following: TSH (thyroid stimulating hormone), total T3 (triiodothyronine) and free T4 (thyroxine), estradiol (major female sex hormone and involved in the regulation of the menstrual reproductive cycle), LH (luteinizing hormone, is a hormone that triggers ovulation in girls if it rises acutely),

FSH (follicle-stimulating hormone, is another hormone that is essential to pubertal development and the function of a woman's ovaries), and testosterone (primary male sex hormone). A number of abnormalities in the endocrine (hormone) system resulting from malnutrition include alteration in growth hormones, elevated secretion of cortisol, and thyroid abnormalities. Levels normalize with nutritional rehabilitation and no medication is generally necessary.

During times of malnutrition, estrogen and testosterone levels may be suppressed, or even undetectable. Insufficient fueling will cause a disturbance in the neuroendocrine system (both the hypothalamic-pituitary-adrenal as well as the hypothalamic-pituitary-gonadal axes) that controls reactions to stress and regulates digestion, the immune system, mood, emotions, sexuality, energy storage, and expenditure. In girls, low estrogen levels will result in missed or irregular periods, (oligomenorrhea), or the complete absence of a period (amenorrhea). Almost one-fourth of female patients with AN develop amenorrhea before the onset of significant weight loss and almost two-thirds during the course of food restriction and weight loss.[8] A full medical workup is necessary to make sure your child's menstrual irregularities aren't due to other hormonal conditions such as polycystic ovarian syndrome (hormonal disorder that can cause irregular menstrual periods), hyperprolactinemia (elevated serum prolactin level), or anatomical abnormalities, to name a few.[9] In boys, where menstrual status is not an option, testosterone levels can be checked.

Regardless of gender, if your child is exhibiting signs of malnutrition, such as cold intolerance, vital-sign instability, or weight loss, your doctor may wish to check your child's hormone levels. However, if your child is menstruating regularly (and is therefore producing sufficient estrogen) or is taking oral contraceptives, checking estrogen levels is not necessary. Hormone levels can be assessed at baseline and tracked throughout treatment. When amenorrhea or a suppressed testosterone level is present, it is recommended to measure hormones every three months as caloric intake and weight improve. More frequent checks usually do not show enough change, and small variations can be easily misinterpreted.

It is important to note that girls with amenorrhea can still ovulate and therefore could become pregnant if sexually active. Women with eating disorders are more likely to have unplanned pregnancies.[10] All sexually active teens, whether menstruating regularly or not, need counseling on using proper contraception. That said, infertility is more common in people struggling with eating disorders.[11] There is a higher rate of pregnancy complications and miscarriages as well as complications of the newborn in women with AN.

There is a direct correlation between weight restoration and improvement of hormone levels such as estradiol and testosterone. Researchers showed that 86 percent of adolescent females resumed menses within six months of achieving a weight at or above 90 percent median body weight for age and height, which translates to approximately the twenty-seventh percentile for BMI.[12] However, about one-third of weight-restored patients with a history of AN remain amenorrheic despite weight restoration.[13] In a chart review looking at the metabolic differences of adolescents who were menstruating compared to those who were not, amenorrheic adolescents had a significantly lower metabolic rate, meaning that on average they were consuming slightly less total calories per day. Amenorrheic adolescents were also found to weigh an average of 8.1 pounds (3.7 kilograms) less than the menstruating group and were consuming less fat.[14]

Our bodies require essential fatty acids (EFAs) to function, which must be obtained directly from dietary sources, including omega-3 fatty acids. Studies have shown that EFA intake can help regulate resumption of menses and the normalization of testosterone, though this hasn't been studied extensively.[15] To reverse the effect of suppressed sex hormones, your child will be encouraged to add more fats and calories to their diet. The extra calories will help to close the energy gap between what their body is burning and what their body is consuming. And the added fats will help their body boost hormones, since fats are required in the synthesis of estrogen and testosterone. See the chart on page 71 for strategies to increase dietary intake of omega-3 fatty acids.

Resumption of menses (ROM)

ROM is a major cornerstone in recovery and is defined by three consecutive menstrual cycles. Menses may be light upon initial return but should resume to what was "normal" for your child prior to the onset of their eating disorder.

ROM requires particular attention from the entire treatment team and is typically met with mixed emotions. On one level, your child is happy that their body is finally getting to a healthy place. But psychologically, it is common for the return of menses to cause an escalation of your child's anxiety, as this signals that they have gained weight and are officially not "dangerously thin." This can be really hard for kids, especially as they are dealing with getting comfortable in a new weight-restored body. At this point, they may assume that they are at a "healthy" weight. However, one period, even though it is encouraging, does not mean your child is ready to stop. The hormonal balance is still fragile, and despite some weight gain, subsequent menstrual cycles can remain irregular. Before making any changes, you and the treatment team should wait until your child has three consecutive periods. It is common to see setbacks during this time due to misinterpretation of what "medical stability" means, and it should be stressed that nutrition must continue in order to achieve full stability and to maintain the recovery process.

A common mistake we see in treatment is for parents and kids to take their foot off the gas at this point. Exhausted from treatment, everyone breathes a sigh of relief, excited to get some good news when the period arrives. We have seen families drop out of treatment prematurely, only to take several steps backward with continued amenorrhea following the return of that one period. As your child nears their goal weight, they may be struggling to accept their new body. Their coping mechanism, the eating disorder, is no longer an option, leaving most feeling more vulnerable than they did when they were malnourished. Your child will need to work with a therapist on accepting their body and finding healthy coping mechanisms. Once periods return to normal, a careful assessment from all members on the team is important to evaluate what your child's future needs are. Some kids might be physically and psychologically ready to test out reducing the

Omega-3 Fatty Acids in the Diet[16]

Fatty fish: Current dietary recommendations are to include fish in your meals at least twice per week. Fish high in omega-3 fats are salmon, albacore tuna (fresh and canned), sardines, lake trout, and mackerel.

Walnuts: Walnuts are an excellent plant-based source of omega-3. Add walnuts to cereal, salads, or muffins. Try walnut oil in salad dressings and sautés, too.

Oils: Replace solid fats such as butter or margarine with oils such as canola and soybean when cooking or baking. It works well for sautéing and stir-frying.

Flaxseed: Add ground flaxseed to breakfast cereal, yogurt, baked goods such as breads and muffins, or mixed dishes and casseroles. Or drizzle flaxseed oil over rice or use it in salad dressing. (The body is unable to break down whole flaxseeds to access the omega-3-containing oil.)

Eggs: Some chickens are given feed that is high in omega-3s so their eggs will contain more as well. When buying eggs, check the package label.

intensity of treatment at this stage, while others will require continued intensive treatment.

Bone mineral density

Peak bone density refers to the bone's maximum strength and density, and is typically achieved during late adolescence. Ninety percent of an adolescent's peak bone density is reached by age eighteen for girls and by age twenty for boys, making adolescence an important time to "invest" in bone health. After peak bone density is reached additional bone accrual is minimal. Later in life, testosterone and estrogen levels drop, causing a natural decline in bone density, often leading to frequent bone breaks. Accruing as much bone density as possible during adolescence is essential for optimizing bone health later in life.

Low bone-mineral density (BMD) is commonly seen in patients with AN as well as BN, and in both boys and girls. Low bone density is one of the most prominent complications of low estrogen (as seen with irregular or absent menses) and low testosterone levels.[17] More than 90 percent of girls with AN have low BMD at one or more sites.[18] Low BMD interferes with the ability for your child to maximize their bone strength and puts them at greater risk for fractures during childhood and adulthood.[19] The duration of amenorrhea caused by low estrogen levels, or the duration of low testosterone levels, is directly correlated to low BMD. Your medical team will assess your child for the risk of low BMD, which can result from poor nutrition including lack of calcium, protein, and vitamin D; low body weight; estrogen deficiency; and/or excessive exercise. The levels of serum 25-hydroxy vitamin D, a hormone that is synthesized in the body and involved in bone metabolism, should be tested and treated if necessary. Normal serum 25-hydroxy vitamin D levels will support bone health and provide other benefits such as immune function, cell growth, and the reduction of inflammation.

The most common method to assess BMD is called dual-energy X-ray absorptiometry (DXA) and is typically recommended once amenorrhea has been present for six months or more.[20] This scan measures the bone-mineral content of a cross-sectional area of bone with a resulting t-score and a z-score. The t-score reflects a young adult population and the z-score reflects an age-matched population. It is important to note that the International Society for Clinical Densitometry (ISCD) recently identified "low bone mass or bone-mineral density" (defined as bone-mineral density z-score greater than or equal to –2.0 SD) as the preferred term for children and adolescents rather than the term osteo-penia. Among adolescent girls, low BMD is more commonly seen in the lumbar spine (lower back), while in boys, low BMD has been shown to be more common at the hip and femoral neck.[21] The amount of radiation is very low at one-tenth the amount of radiation in a standard chest X-ray.

You might be wondering if adding the birth control pill (supple-mented hormones that allow your child to menstruate) would be ben-eficial here. As it turns out, the birth control pill and other hormone therapies don't fix the bone issues associated with malnutrition as currently practiced, though research continues to be done in this area. The biggest predictor of improved bone density is actually an improved body weight.[22] And further, once on the pill and menstruating the child often thinks "they're fine" and "done." The act of menstruating, even though artificially induced, can then discourage the child from continu-ing to work on an improved diet. The weight at which the body resumes menstruation is an important marker for recovery. Without that nat-ural marker, a person's goal weight becomes less clear. Those actively seeking the return of menstruation are motivated to work harder to get their period back, a clear goal that is a reward for their efforts. That said, if someone is on the pill, vital signs and nutritional assessment can provide useful information.

Unfortunately, low BMD in both boys and girls may not be entirely reversible, despite optimal medical and nutritional interventions.[23] Your medical team will likely recommend an annual DXA scan to monitor for any changes and will adjust the type and amount of authorized activity for your child depending on the results. Ways to treat low BMD include:

- Weight restoration
- Normalization of hormones, with ROM for females
- Optimal calcium intake (1,300 milligrams per day)
- Optimal vitamin D intake (600 international units per day)
- Treatment of vitamin D deficiency
- Weight-bearing physical activity (if medically approved)

Brain Changes

Imaging studies show that there is visible loss of brain substance in malnourished individuals with AN, also called cerebral atrophy. The findings are so profound, in fact, that the MRI of an anorexic brain can look comparable to that of an individual with Alzheimer's disease.[24] While your child might show a surprising degree of accomplishments at school and in daily life, we see children develop difficulty concentrating and with retention of information over time. Weight gain is not immediately associated with improvement in MRI brain scans, especially of the gray matter. Note that brain imaging is not used for regular monitoring.

Boys and Eating Disorders

In general, we have limited information and studies about boys affected with eating disorders, but some studies suggest that they account for 10 percent of all diagnosed eating-disorder cases, with a higher prevalence found among gay men than among straight men.[25] While there is not an easily identifiable physiological marker of malnutrition in boys as with menses in girls, there are several medical complications that occur. Boys naturally have a lower percentage of body fat and higher muscle mass than girls and often present to the medical provider with more severe weight loss, clinical, and laboratory findings. Laboratory tests should include serum testosterone levels to assess hormone levels, which are typically low in the context of malnutrition. Various studies suggest that risk of mortality for boys with eating disorders is higher than for girls. Men with eating disorders often suffer from additional conditions, such as depression, substance abuse disorders, and anxiety.

Metabolism

During malnutrition, one's metabolic rate slows down as an adaptive response to starvation. Resting energy expenditure (REE; defined as the amount of calories the body needs over twenty-four hours to perform its basic bodily functions while at rest) decreases and may be 50 to 75 percent of what would be expected for their age, height, weight, and gender.[26] The metabolic rate after prolonged food restriction or irregular food intake will be significantly lower than average initially and will quickly increase during the refeeding process.[27] This requires constant adjustments to ensure continued and safe metabolic recovery, which can take several months, even years, and requires a multidisciplinary team approach. Medical fragility can last for a prolonged period of time and can continue even after full metabolic recovery is achieved.

Body Composition

During the weight restoration process, weight is often distributed more centrally to protect internal organs but typically disperses to the arms and legs with time. This is also the normal progression of weight gain during adolescence with hormonal changes and the development of a more adult figure. You should not worry about your child's weight distribution at this stage of recovery and seek guidance from the therapist as needed to facilitate healthy conversations about the weight gain process with your child.

Timeline of When Medical Complications Resolve[28]

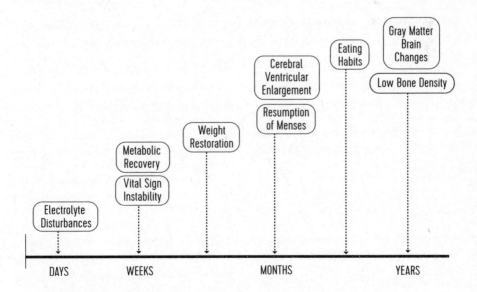

The Initial Medical Assessment

Depending on the background and training of the medical provider you choose for the initial assessment and follow-up care of your child, your visit can vary in length and structure. Only a few medical subspecialists exist in the field of adolescent eating disorders. Training can be acquired through a fellowship and board certification in adolescent medicine with a focus in adolescents with eating disorders. Often the primary care provider takes on the medical management of an adolescent with an eating disorder. There are guidelines available on how to assess for medical stability in this population through specialized treatment centers and online (see the website for the Academy for Eating Disorders, aedweb.org).

During any medical visit (initial or follow-up) you can expect the medical professional to check the following:

- Your child's weight and height while in a gown (ideally blind, for example by stepping onto the scale backward) and after urination (supervised with the door cracked, to listen for interfering behaviors).
- Blood pressure and heart rate after lying down (supine position) for five minutes in a quiet room, and after standing up for two minutes.
- A urinalysis, which measures hydration (specific gravity); acid/base status (pH testing), for information on recent vomiting; presence of ketones, which is a sign of starvation; and signs of infection in the urine to name a few. (Many providers include a mandatory urine toxicology screen as well, to monitor for any drug use that can interfere with treatment.)
- An EKG (electrocardiogram) to measure electrical activity of the heart.

Other things you can expect after, or prior to the visit:

- Baseline blood work is usually requested. Blood work generally includes a complete blood count (CBC); comprehensive metabolic panel (CMP), including magnesium and phosphorus level; thyroid hormones; pancreatic enzymes (amylase and lipase); vitamin D level; and sedimentation rate (ESR).

- If your child has lost their period for more than three months (known as secondary amenorrhea; primary amenorrhea refers to someone who has not had their period by age fifteen) and is not taking hormones such as oral contraceptive pills, an estradiol level and other hormone levels may be ordered.
- If your child has prolonged secondary amenorrhea of more than six months, a bone density scan (DXA) will be recommended. Recommendations for DXA scans in males vary.

Table for Eating-Disorders Medical Assessment

WHAT TO ASSESS	SPECIAL CONSIDERATIONS FOR EATING DISORDERS
Weight, height	In gown, after urination, blind
Heart rate	Lying down for 5 minutes, standing for 2 minutes
Blood pressure	Lying down for 5 minutes, standing for 2 minutes
Temperature	Under the tongue
Urinalysis (specific gravity, pH, ketones)	Supervised with door cracked
Urine toxicology (optional)	Supervised with door cracked
Electrical activity of heart	EKG can be done in office
Blood: CBC, CMP, vit. D, ESR, thyroid	Can be done prior to initial medical visit
Estradiol level	If amenorrheic for 3 months
Bone-mineral density: DXA	If amenorrheic for 6 months

During the initial medical visit the provider should meet with you and your child separately as well as together. This often provides more information, as you and your child may not be comfortable sharing as much information with the provider when in the same room. If your child is eighteen years or older, he or she will need to give consent to the provider to meet and to share any information with you. In addition to a complete medical history, the provider will assess for eating-disorder behaviors, exercise, menstrual history, current medications or supplements, and trauma, and obtain a psychosocial history. A review of CDC growth charts that have tracked your child's weight and height since birth is helpful for the provider and would ideally be submitted prior to the initial assessment. Any details about childhood development and eating habits can add valuable information.

The next part of the visit is the physical exam and is usually completed without the parent present. In addition to a regular head-to-toe check, the medical provider will focus on the following areas that can be particularly affected by an eating disorder: skin, hair, nails, lymph nodes, glands, cardiovascular system, gastrointestinal system, respiratory system, and Tanner staging (scale of sexual development). An initial consultation and assessment might last anywhere from one to three hours. Your provider should communicate findings of the assessment to you and will give recommendations about the next best steps. These might include blood work, bone-density scans or other tests, and often include referrals for therapists, dietitians, psychiatrists, an occupational therapist, or other medical subspecialists such as an endocrinologist or a cardiologist. The medical provider will typically schedule follow-up visits ranging from weekly to every few months. If your child is medically unstable, your provider might recommend immediate medical hospitalization or another higher level of care (residential treatment, partial hospitalization, or intensive outpatient treatment). Please follow the medical advice you receive closely as this will assure the best outcome possible.

Assessing the Degree of Malnutrition and Setting Weight Goals

The first step in deciding a weight goal for your child is to assess the degree to which your child is malnourished. This can be easily assessed by your child's medical provider. Your provider will first take your child's height and weight, and then calculate your child's body mass index (BMI; weight in kilograms divided by height in meters squared). The

List of criteria for medical hospitalization[29]

- Less than 75 percent median body mass index for age and sex
- Dehydration
- Hypoglycemia
- Electrolyte disturbance
- EKG abnormalities
- Physiological instability
  - Severe bradycardia (heart rate fewer than fifty beats per minute at daytime; fewer than 45 beats per minute at night)
  - Hypotension or low blood pressure (less than 90/45 mm Hg)
  - Hypothermia (body temperature less than 96 degrees Fahrenheit, 35.6 degrees Celsius)
  - Orthostatic increase in pulse (greater than twenty beats per minute) or decrease in blood pressure (greater than 20 mm Hg systolic or greater than 10 mm Hg diastolic)
- Arrested growth and development
- Failure of outpatient treatment
- Acute food refusal
- Uncontrollable binging and purging
- Acute medical complications of malnutrition (for example fainting, seizures, cardiac failure, pancreatitis)
- Comorbid psychiatric or medical condition that prohibits or limits appropriate outpatient treatment (e.g., severe depression, suicidal ideation, obsessive compulsive disorder, type 1 diabetes mellitus)

BMI takes into account the relationship between height and weight. Your pediatrician will then plot these values on the Centers for Disease Control and Prevention (CDC) growth charts, used for children and adolescents up to the age of twenty, and compare your child's measurements to a reference population. Current percent of median BMI can then be calculated (your child's BMI divided by the fiftieth percentile BMI for your child's age and sex, multiplied by one hundred), and then compared again to the reference population. Percent median BMI, along with the percent of weight loss and changes in BMI percentiles, are several ways your medical provider can assess malnutrition. Mild, moderate, and severe malnutrition is characterized as a percentage of the determined goal weight.

Of note, your child's weight should be assessed in a medical gown after urinating. This helps to keep weight checks consistent and makes it more difficult for your child to manipulate their weight. The weight should be shared with you; however, there are two schools of thought regarding whether the weight on the scale should be shared with your child. In family-based treatment, therapists often share and discuss the weight openly, seeing this as a chance to reduce fear around a number and acclimate the child to the weight-gain process. On the other hand, hearing the numbers and the trajectory can be so distressing for a child with an eating disorder that providers may wish to keep the weight private, until the child feels ready to hear the number. Tolerance to seeing the weight does improve as your child reaches their goal weight, though kids may often struggle with the numbers long after they are recovered. Keeping weight a secret for too long can also backfire, leaving the child shocked if they stumble across it one day. An open discussion with the treatment team is recommended to understand how each child feels and what would best support them.

Setting Weight Goals

Setting weight goals for an adolescent struggling with an eating disorder is both an art and a science. Your child's treatment team will determine a

Horizontal Growth Curve Indicating Weight Plateau
During a Time When a Child Should Have Been Gaining

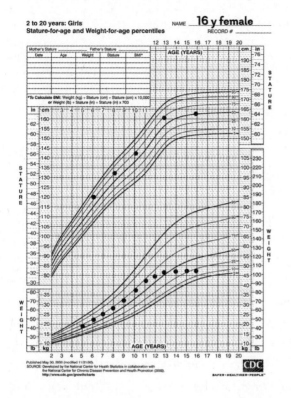

goal weight by using BMI charts as well as your child's historical growth curves. The recommended "treatment goal weight" is usually a range of weights where medical complications are expected to resolve. In this goal weight range, the preoccupations with food, weight, and shape are usually less, though still may be present to some extent.

While not every child needs to gain weight, most of them usually do in order to treat the physiological complications of their eating disorder. Adolescents are often considered moving targets, and a good goal weight in one year may change the following year as they grow. This can be hard for kids (or parents) who may say, "But she *never* weighed more than 103 pounds, why should she be 110 now?" But if your child stayed 103 pounds from ages twelve through fifteen, their growth curve would actually look more like a horizontal line, rather than a curve, which would jeopardize your child's ability to grow and develop normally.

According to the recent position statement from the Society for Adolescent Health and Medicine, "during a period of growth, goal weights should be assessed every three–six months."[1] Quite simply, as kids grow they need to weigh more. And sometimes, they might need to increase their weight first to stimulate growth, especially if growth had been delayed due to malnutrition. It is imperative that you and your child understand that weight goals set for your adolescent are ever changing and that your child will likely need to continue to gain weight into their late adolescence.

Medical providers can use median BMI to set weight goals; however, that value is based on a reference population and doesn't take into account your child's historical growth patterns. To set a customized weight goal, the medical provider will obtain and review your child's growth curves, which will help describe your child's earlier pattern of growth prior to the onset of their eating disorder. Your child's growth curves are their body's blueprint, unique to them, and your medical provider will evaluate these growth curves to determine what percentile they historically tracked along for weight, height, and body mass index (BMI). This can be a valuable tool for estimating weight goals. Height charts are also useful to determine whether your child's linear growth has been compromised through malnutrition. Your child's growth curves, with data collected over their lifetime, can provide a more customized range for where your child's weight should fall for optimal health.

Case Example: Sahil

Sahil is a thirteen-year-old boy diagnosed with anorexia nervosa at age twelve and a half. In talking with his parents, they point out that Sahil was previously a "chubby" boy and they are unsure what his healthy weight range should be. They share that he was told by his pediatrician at age twelve that he was "overweight" and that he needed to eat more fruit and vegetables, increase activity, and play fewer computer games. Sahil is a "rule follower," per his parents, and when he heard that message he immediately started following the doctor's recommendations. In about three months' time, he lost five pounds, which his parents and the doctor thought was great. Unfortunately, this pattern continued, and by the time six months had passed, he had lost fifteen pounds, resulting in a fainting episode during PE class at school. What his parents and doctor didn't see was how obsessive, rigid with food, and compulsive with exercise he had become. What started out with good intentions spiraled quickly out of control to a dangerous place.

In looking at Sahil's growth charts, the treatment team noticed his weight had historically plotted along the seventy-fifth percentile until age twelve. It then dropped to the sixty-fifth percentile after he started losing weight. By the time Sahil was diagnosed with anorexia nervosa, his weight had dropped to the fiftieth percentile for his age. Of note, a weight at the fiftieth percentile "looks average." So his weight might appear to be a normal weight, yet Sahil was clearly suffering medically and psychologically at this point. His linear growth was also affected. While he had previously tracked along the seventy-fifth percentile in height for his age, the rapid weight loss compromised Sahil's growth, and by age thirteen, his height was tracking along the fiftieth percentile. Crossing percentiles on a growth curve or premature plateaus in height are often markers of malnutrition in kids and are highly abnormal in young teenagers, especially boys. Fortunately, at Sahil's young age, he likely has room to catch up in height growth with strong nutritional rehabilitation.

Sahil's parents asked the treatment team what his ideal body weight is. The treatment team used standard measures as well as the growth chart to determine this range. The team told the family they could evaluate how things looked when Sahil gained some weight, improved his diet, and reached around the sixty-fifth percentile. But even at this interim goal weight range, there were still signs of malnutrition. Despite gaining some weight and eating more, Sahil's heart rate and body temperature continued to be quite low. He was still obsessive about food, and it then became clear to the team and his parents that they needed to shift the goal weight range back up to the seventy-fifth percentile, where his weight had always been.

The team discussed with Sahil's parents that weight is only one marker of health and that it would be critical to his long-term health and chances for catching up in height to get him back on his natural growth curve while working on developing healthy behaviors with food and activity. The team explained to his parents that there is a wide range of what is considered "healthy" and that with the exception of too much screen time, Sahil had otherwise been healthy when he was at the seventy-fifth percentile. At that time, he likely would have benefited from a few minor lifestyle changes without need for weight loss. Not surprisingly, when Sahil eventually reached the seventy-fifth percentile, his vital signs normalized, his mood improved, and he became more social again. "He's back!" his parents exclaimed. They hadn't seen the real Sahil in months.

It takes many pieces of data for the treatment team to determine optimal weight goals. In girls who stopped menstruating as a result of malnutrition, the resumption of menses is a strong indicator of complete weight restoration. But what about individuals who never lost their period during malnutrition? Or what about boys? Clinicians should look at the whole individual and take into account a child's growth curves and growth trajectory, blood work, puberty-related development, as well as menstrual status if applicable.

In addition, there are often psychological indicators that help determine when your child is in a healthy weight range: your child may seem like their "normal" self again; they may have stopped negotiating about food; they may be more sociable and want to go out to eat at their old favorite restaurants; and they are likely no longer constantly thinking about food and weight. And while there is little research about the psychological benefits of weight restoration, these results are commonly seen in practice.[2]

Trust Your Medical Provider

The medical complications associated with eating disorders can seem daunting, especially if this is your first time dealing with one. The priority is making sure your child is safe and medically stable throughout this process (and if not, that you seek recommendations from the treatment team). You will need the help of a medical provider to sort through all of the medical complications of your child's eating disorder and you should not be afraid to ask questions. The good news is that almost all complications are reversible with renourishment. Food—not pills or supplements—is the remedy. Your child's fatigue, irritability, dizziness, orange fingers, hair loss—to name a few—can improve dramatically once your child is consuming a sufficient amount of nutrients. So while it may seem disheartening to see your child so physically and emotionally fragile, there is hope. Implementation of the Plate-by-Plate approach alongside FBT will help your child heal as quickly as possible.

CHAPTER 5

——◗▶——

To Exercise or Not

Managing Athletes, Exercise, and Compulsive Movement

APPROXIMATELY **50** PERCENT of those struggling with an eating disorder also struggle with compulsive exercise[1] and there is a higher incidence of eating disorders present among athletes.[2] Sports are a large part of almost all households and can be integral in helping kids to develop coordination, social skills, leadership skills, and respect for others. Physical activity helps to improve mood, reduce stress and anxiety, increase energy, longevity, and can help improve body image. However, in the context of an eating disorder, the benefits of exercise can backfire, intensifying one's preoccupation with food, weight, and shape, while increasing obsessiveness and compulsiveness around the need to exercise. Frequent physical activity, paired with a limited or restricted diet, can compromise a child's medical status—increasing their risk for injury, or worse, hospitalization. The decision of whether to allow your child to exercise or not should be carefully considered by the entire treatment team, who can assess medical, psychological, and nutritional readiness.

RED-S: Relative Energy Deficiency in Sport

You might be thinking to yourself, "Wait a minute, I thought exercise was supposed to be *good* for you?" It can be, however, exercising while not eating enough can harm the body and dramatically worsen performance. A caloric imbalance, whether intentional, due to an eating disorder, or unintentional—due to being too busy or having too high of a training load—can cause negative effects among every system in the body. There will be negative effects on your child's endocrine system (reduction of hormones), growth and development, metabolism, gastrointestinal system, bones, and cardiovascular system, to name a few (as discussed in chapter 4). Athletes who are not properly fueling may be slower, weaker, more prone to injury, irritable, depressed, and have decreased endurance. This is ironic, given their initial goal of achieving health and excelling at their sport.

Researchers have described a syndrome known as relative energy deficiency in sport (RED-S), which highlights the effects that even a small energy imbalance has on both men and women. Eating slightly less than what a person's body requires, whether intentional or unintentional, can cause impairments in almost every area of the body, notably disturbances in a person's menstrual cycle, bone health, immune function, and vital signs.[3] RED-S updates the female athlete triad, which previously described a triad of reduced energy availability, reduced bone health, and suppressed menstrual function in girls. Similar to RED-S, the female athlete triad highlights the negative effects of eating too little for one's energy output, yet RED-S captures the deleterious effects on many body systems, rather than just on menstruation and bone health.

An athlete experiencing RED-S may notice they miss a period, or that they are feeling sluggish and weak, and this often propels them to seek help. Again, an athlete may get into a mismatched energy state by accident, simply by training too hard or too long, without carefully matching their intake of energy (by way of food). This is common in sports with long training schedules and for someone training for endurance events like a marathon or an IRONMAN distance triathlon.

Prevalence of Amenorrhea Among Female Athletes[4]

- 10 to 15 percent of female athletes
- 67 percent of elite female athletes
- 12 percent of swimmers and cyclists
- 20 percent of vigorous exercisers
- 44 percent of ballet dancers
- 50 percent of female triathletes
- 51 percent of endurance runners

The energy imbalance is something that can be calculated by a registered dietitian who specializes in both sports nutrition and the treatment of eating disorders. The dietitian may also be a board-certified specialist in sports dietetics (CSSD). They can assess how much your child is eating, how much they are burning, and determine exactly whether an energy imbalance exists. This may not be "exact" but will provide a general overview of your child's overall needs. Correcting an energy deficit, simply by training less, eating more, or both, reverses most of the associated complications and improves performance. Specifically, adding a supplemental shake, adding more rest days, increasing total caloric intake, and improving dietary practices in general can be helpful in closing the energy gap.[5]

For some athletes, once the energy imbalance is identified, they are motivated to close the gap between energy expenditure and energy intake. They come to realize that eating more will help them fix many of the medical and psychological side effects they have been experiencing. For others, they may carry a fear that adding more food will negatively affect their weight, their performance, or how they feel while competing. It is here that we educate about the effects of RED-S, as well as how one's metabolic rate will increase with the increasing caloric intake. As a person increases their caloric intake, their body begins to burn more calories. This results in an improved metabolism, which is connected to improved energy, endurance, stamina, appetite, performance, and recovery from exercise.

Balanced versus compulsive exercise

Similar to eating a healthy diet, being fit and exercising regularly attracts praise and admiration in our society. All too often, however, these lifestyle changes can be accompanied by an eating disorder as one's relationship with exercise may shift from being mindful, balanced, and healthy to being all-consuming, obsessive, and harmful. Approximately 39 to 48 percent of individuals with eating disorders exercise compulsively.[6] You should be on the lookout for abnormal exercise behaviors such as a child who "can't stop" or feels guilty for taking a day off from exercise, which may signal a greater problem. Someone who has an unhealthy relationship with exercise may be unable to or uncomfortable with sitting still; they might stand while watching TV or movies, pace around the house, climb up and down stairs multiple times, or sit in certain ways at the table so as to contract their abdominal muscles or engage their leg muscles. For example, a compulsive exerciser might do ten squats every time they pick something off the ground, or study while in a "plank" pose.

Someone struggling with compulsive exercise may run around the block while walking the dog, sneak YouTube exercise videos in at night, or run in place in the shower. Some individuals tell themselves they can only eat if they can exercise, or punish themselves for eating "something bad" with a certain number of compensatory exercises. Teens who have developed a concerning relationship with exercise may train while injured or sick, or lose interest in their once-beloved sport and opt for something more intense.

They may put themselves in danger by exercising in extreme conditions (heat waves, freezing temperatures), very early-morning or late-night hours. Additionally, there may be a high level of anxiety associated with missed practices or training sessions that can result in compensatory behaviors (e.g., restricting calories) in an effort to alleviate emotional distress. One teen was upset when her coach had canceled practices due to the record high 110-degree day. Fearful that her "muscles would disappear" she ran out in the heat anyway, eventually ending up in the emergency room with severe dehydration and unintentional vomiting. Safety and health must be prioritized over exercise routine.

Case Example: Jacob

For months, Jacob's parents had been yelling at him to walk the dog, but Jacob had refused, saying he was "too busy" or "had too much schoolwork." One day, Jacob announced that he would be in charge of all the dog walking every day. Karen, Jacob's mother, was thrilled but puzzled. She couldn't help but wonder, "Why is Jacob suddenly so interested in walking the dog?" A few weeks later, Karen found Jacob halfway down the street when she was running an errand and was surprised to find Jacob really sweaty, out of breath, and with his face flushed red. She knew walking the dog wouldn't make him that sweaty. That moment was a turning point for Jacob's parents. They began to wonder, "What has Jacob really been doing all those times while he was walking the dog, and more important, why was he hiding it?"

Being observant is important in this process, as, ultimately, you can best recognize a change in your child's behavior and can address concerning issues proactively before they further intensify and compromise your child's health. Compulsive exercise can be scary and have far-reaching consequences that can have serious medical, psychological, and emotional ramifications. Excessive exercise puts an individual at increased risk for injury (overuse injuries, stress fractures, muscle pulls or tears). It can cause a loss of bone density, the absence of one's menstrual cycle, persistent muscle soreness, fatigue, and sluggishness.

Case Example: Leora

Years of amenorrhea had caught up with Leora. She had stress fractures in both legs and was told by the orthopedist to take a break from running. But she couldn't adhere to those guidelines, and instead, took up biking. She biked for more than sixty minutes a day, despite being underweight, medically fragile, and injured. She was in a lot of pain. Her stress fracture got worse, until finally, her legs swelled up, causing her to need to go to the emergency room.

Underfueling, while being unable to take a break during injury, quickly puts someone at medical risk. For Leora, her ER visit was a turning point, a moment when her parents realized, "Okay, something is wrong here."

It is important to understand the intent or motivation to exercise. Exercise that is completed to focus on altering weight and shape or "burning calories" should be of concern. Instead, teens should focus on the benefits that come with exercise, such as improved energy, mood, and sleep. Exercise should be enjoyable and energizing, not completely exhausting or painful. In a healthy relationship with exercise an individual should be able to vary the intensity of workouts, meaning that training can occur at a lower intensity some of the time and more intensely at others. Someone who is compulsively exercising may only know and exhibit one gear—high intensity, or near maximum effort—during workouts. They may struggle with a fierce adherence to rigid exercise routines, whereas those who exercise mindfully can be more flexible. For example, if it's cold and raining outside, a balanced exerciser may decide to skip a run and opt for a cup of tea and a good book by the fire. Conversely, a compulsive exerciser will go out in the cold and rain, perhaps in the early-morning hours when it's still dark out, to run miles and miles anyway. While following a balanced diet, an individual who exercises moderately will often see incremental performance gains, whereas an individual who exercises compulsively will likely experience a decline in performance over time.

> ### Case Example: Serena
>
> Serena was a seventeen-year-old volleyball player, heading off to a Division I school to play volleyball on scholarship. She was so excited about this opportunity that she began training two hours in the morning (five to seven, before school) and two hours in the evening. She was barely eating and became obsessed with "getting toned." She was shocked when her high school coach benched her midgame. She was the one heading to a Division 1 school on scholarship! He told her she looked pale, tired, and "gassed." He asked what was wrong, was she injured? She was not the player he knew.

For all athletes, rest is important. Those struggling with compulsive exercise will say that rest is unnecessary or a waste of time. Oftentimes, they perceive rest days as being lazy or unproductive. However, rest helps the muscular, nervous, and immune systems recover and strengthen. Rest helps athletes minimize soreness, inflammation, and illness while allowing the body to rebuild and prepare for the next day. On days of rest, the body may not engage in exercise, but it is very active while healing and repairing itself. Taking rest days optimizes performance. Collegiate athletes and professional athletes often do not train seven days a week—they are careful to prevent overuse injuries, since they depend on their body for their livelihood. Several rest days per week are recommended, even for elite athletes. In fact, the harder and more intense the workouts are, the more rest days per week are recommended to recover. Nick Paparesta, head athletic trainer for Major League Baseball's Oakland Athletics, recommends that young athletes, who train intensely, get three days of rest per week. "Rest helps with the lengthening of muscular fibers after exercise, which in turn will allow athletes to have better muscle gains moving forward," he says.

	MINDFUL/HEALTHY EXERCISE	COMPULSIVE EXERCISE
GOAL	To challenge oneself and engage in a variety of activities that are enjoyable and energizing	To alter one's appearance and/or negative discomfort
PERFORMANCE OUTCOMES	Incremental gains	Plateaus/decreases
MIND-SET	Work hard/rest hard	Move to move/rest is unnecessary
PACE	Athletes have many gears, including very slow, and they use all of them	One gear only: fast/intense
ROLE	Exercise is only one part of identity, and it is enjoyable	Exercise is the *only* form of identity, and activity is mandatory
APPROACH	Flexible and adaptable	Rigid
APPROACH	Curious/open to new information	Close-minded
APPROACH	Resourceful, driven, and rational	Compulsive and anxious
INJURY	Modify due to illness and injury	Train through illness and injury

Reprinted with permission from Kate Bennett, PsyD, Sport Psychologist (2017)

Including meditation, massage, hot baths, acupuncture, and gentle stretching or yoga in an exercise plan can help improve the body's recovery and healing time. For any child who is recovering from an eating disorder, rest days should be mandatory and exercise should be contingent on meeting their nutritional needs in addition to other treatment targets. The scope of the exercise plan and the number of rest days can be determined by the treatment team and might change over the course of treatment.

When to Bench Your Child from Exercise

Medical considerations

To ensure your child is safe during exercise, they must be medically stable. If your child is not medically stable, there is a greater risk of dizziness, fainting, fatigue, injury, and sudden death. To be medically stable, your child's physician will assess a variety of factors, such as your child's weight and vital signs, including pulse and blood pressure, and body temperature. (For more information, see chapter 4.) The child should be greater than 85 percent median BMI for their age. They should have stable vitals that include: a heart rate over fifty beats per minute during the day and over forty-five beats per minute at night, a blood pressure that is over ninety millimeters mercury systolic, and a body temperature above 96 degrees Fahrenheit (35.6 degrees Celsius).[7] Additionally, there shouldn't be large changes in vital-sign readings when taken in various positions, such as from lying down to sitting up to standing. A large jump, such as a change in pulse over twenty beats per minute or a systolic change in blood pressure over 20 mm Hg, is considered orthostasis, a medical complication of malnutrition that can significantly increase risk if or when the body is stressed via exercise.

If your child is deemed medically unstable, it is recommended that your child seek adequate treatment (possibly hospitalization) and abstain from all exercise. Many medical instabilities can be reversed by ceasing all exercise and increasing fuel with close monitoring by a treatment team. Additionally, a higher level of care, such as a partial-hospitalization program or an intensive outpatient treatment program, may be needed to provide increased support to contain compulsive exercise or other compensatory behaviors that contribute to medical instability.

Nutritional considerations

Exercise increases a person's total caloric requirements. In order for a child to be allowed to exercise, they will need to be able to increase their intake to account for their increased energy expenditure. In a child who is avoiding snacks, avoiding meals, hiding or throwing away foods, and fearful of food in general, it is unlikely that they can take in enough fuel. Running three to four miles a day at cross-country practice, in the absence of a diet that adequately meets their increased energy requirements, generally causes weight loss and a decline in vital sign stability. Even small amounts of exercise can make it more difficult for your child to meet their energy needs. In addition, your child should be compliant with the nutritional increases recommended as their exercise program changes.

Psychological considerations

Whether or not your child is benched from exercise, your child should work on exploring other coping strategies besides exercise to help manage their emotions. They should be encouraged to speak with a therapist about developing a list of skills to use in the absence of exercise and understand that, in the short-term, there might not be a coping behavior that will provide similar positive emotional and physical benefits that exercise has provided. You can help facilitate the development of these skills by offering alternatives to exercise. Using other strategies, such as painting or playing the violin, is helpful for creating a more balanced approach to exercise in the long run. Athletes who rely solely on exercise for their self-worth, identity, or for coping strategies, often struggle enormously when they get injured or cut from the team. The following is a list of restful activities your child can and should be encouraged to engage in if they are "benched," or even to help create a more balanced relationship with exercise:

- Reading
- Art
- Movies
- Scenic drives with the family
- Self-care: facials, manicure/pedicures, massage, bubble baths
- Board games
- Computer/video games
- Listening to music
- Playing an instrument (drums and marching band are the exception here, as both can be quite active)
- Journaling

As your child's food and exercise become more balanced, you should see a reduction in the perseveration around exercise. Initially, kids may present as not being able to think about or talk about anything else. They will obsess about why they should be allowed to exercise and will fight with the team to let them do more. When kids can finally take a step back and stop obsessing about when and how much they can exercise, you can trust that their eating disorder has receded enough for them to implement a balanced exercise program.

Criteria to Be Cleared for Exercise

Medical criteria

A medical professional is necessary to assess the following.

- Greater than 85 percent median body weight for their age
- Pulse (heart rate) greater than fifty beats per minute and above forty-five beats per minute at night
- Systolic blood pressure over 90 mm Hg
- No orthostatic[*] changes noted
- Normal body temperature, above 96 degrees Fahrenheit (35.6 degrees Celsius)
- Normal blood work, including electrolytes
- Adequate hydration (can test urine specific gravity levels, 1.010–1.020 is considered normal)
- Safe to proceed from an injury-healing standpoint

Nutritional criteria

- Compliant with nutrition recommendations
- Agreeable to nutrition increases, if necessary

Psychological criteria

- Compliant with treatment goals
- Able to stick to the agreed-upon duration, intensity, and frequency of exercise
- Agrees to take a rest day
- Utilizes other coping strategies besides exercise
- Reduced perseveration around exercise

*Orthostasis refers to changes in pulse and blood pressure when a person goes from lying down, to sitting up, to standing. Change in pulse over twenty beats per minute or a blood pressure with a change of more than 10 mm Hg is considered orthostatic and means the heart has been compromised. Again, this is assessed by a medical provider.

Case Example: Kara

Kara was pulled from cross-country practice when she continued to lose weight over three consecutive medical appointments. Her vitals were trending downward, and the doctor was concerned about her fragile medical status, especially when paired with her lack of compliance with nutrition recommendations. Kara cried in the doctor's office that day, and her parents felt torn; they hated seeing Kara so upset and knew exercise would calm her down, yet they understood that if Kara kept eating that way and exercising that much, her vital signs would worsen and she would quickly end up in the hospital. Kara's parents agreed to pull her from cross-country, yet they still allowed her to walk the dog each day, bike to and from school, and hike with her friends on the weekend. Despite stopping cross-country, at the next medical visit, Kara's heart rate had worsened. Her pulse was forty-eight beats per minute in the doctor's office; she was orthostatic by pulse (change of twenty-four beats per minute upon standing), and her body temperature showed she was hypothermic. The doctor recommended hospitalization at that point.

When someone is benched from exercise, it typically means their body needs time to heal—like a broken leg, which may require some time on crutches. All exercise counts as energy expenditure and translates to calories burned that will require your child to eat more. Even if your child has been pulled from their team sport, or main form of exercise, you should carefully consider the total amount of movement that your child is doing. Especially if medically fragile, it is important to cut back where possible. If your child was recovering from mononucleosis, they most likely wouldn't be traveling all over town, working long shifts at their after-school job, or spending large amounts of time away from the house. Resting due to your child's eating disorder is no different; your child is sick and needs rest in order to heal. Some areas you may wish to consider:

- Is your child walking or biking to school?
- Do they walk the dog?
- Are they constantly pacing up and down the stairs?
- Have you checked their internet history for exercise videos?
- Have you observed your child exercising in their room?
- Does your child participate in PE class at school?
- Are they volunteering or working all day, and standing on their feet for many hours?
- Is your child gone for long periods of time without you knowing where they are, or what they are doing?

Kids and parents often struggle with this idea of stopping exercise and eating more. "You want me to sit out of soccer *and* eat more?" There is an intense fear that without training, their body will "turn to mush" and that they will only gain fat. However, as a malnourished individual gains weight, they gain in many areas of the body. It's not just fat. Weight gain occurs in the muscles, bones, brain, liver, and kidneys. In chapter 4 you read about how several systems in the body shut down due to malnutrition, and yet with nourishment and weight gain, each one of these systems turns back on. This helps to improve energy, strength, and cognitive function.

What Can You Do?

As a parent, you can intervene by providing close supervision of your child and their activity patterns. Interrupting random sit-ups, or squats, and insisting they sit while watching TV or doing homework can help them stop these behaviors. If your child cannot stay still at night while you are sleeping, you may consider sleeping in their room or installing a motion sensor in their bedroom. If your child does not respond to the limits you set, they may need additional help. In some cases, psychiatric medications are recommended and are currently being explored for the treatment of compulsive exercise. Recognizing that these behaviors are not healthy for your child and seeking the help of a trained professional is the first step in helping your child to recover and eventually rebuild their relationship with exercise.

Talking through what "balanced exercise" means with your child and modeling it at home will help your child heal. Rest days should be nonnegotiable, as they are even for elite athletes, and you should help your child learn how to implement other restful activities on those days.

You may struggle initially with having to reduce or stop your child's exercise program, but ultimately, this will help your child recover more quickly, both medically and psychologically. It might be unfathomable to your child, but taking a break from training, improving nutrition, and gaining weight (increased muscle mass, bone density, and cardio-vascular function) are the keys to becoming a stronger, more consistent athlete who will be less susceptible to injury. Benching your child from exercise is certainly not easy but it is guaranteed to help your child heal.

PART II

The Plate-by-Plate Approach

CHAPTER 6

Refeeding Your Child
and Achieving a
Balanced Plate

Phase 1 of FBT

Assessing Your Child's Plate: Then and Now

BEFORE BEGINNING THE Plate-by-Plate approach, it's important to assess your child's diet. If you are already working with a registered dietitian, this is something the dietitian will do initially with you in order to get a sense of how your child is eating. If you are not yet working with a dietitian, this seven-day "snapshot" will be a helpful starting point. You may think you know how your child eats, but there is something very powerful about seeing it on paper, meal after meal. Keep a seven-day record, and log every breakfast, lunch, dinner, and snack.

While you might not yet know exactly how much food your child requires each day, you will likely have a sense that their current diet is insufficient. (We don't expect parents to count calories; if you are working with a dietitian, this is something the dietitian can assess.) Parents are often keenly aware of areas in their child's diet that are inadequate. For example, their child may have sworn off carbs, or decided to be gluten-free and vegan. Using the seven-day records you have filled out,

Daily Food Record

MEAL	1	2	3	4	5	6	7
BREAKFAST							
SNACK							
LUNCH							
SNACK							
DINNER							
SNACK							

take the following assessment questionnaire to gain more insight into your child's current and past eating patterns. Is your child eating meals and snacks consistently? Can you list the carbohydrates, proteins, fruits, vegetables, fats, and dairy foods that your child is currently eating? A kid will often say, "I'm eating fine; I had a great dinner last night." Or they may share that they had a cookie at school, and therefore they are "fine" and don't have any concerns with sugar. In order to truly understand your child's dietary patterns, you will need to assess whether your child is eating these foods consistently and normally rather than to prove a point.

Assess Your Child's Diet

These questions will provide a quick snapshot of areas that might need improvement in your child's diet. We will come back to this list later on and use it as a road map for the work that needs to be done to best support your child's recovery.

Is your child eating three meals and a few snacks each day?

Are they skipping meals, and if so, how many breakfasts, lunches, or dinners per week are they actually eating?

My child is eating _____ out of seven breakfasts

My child is eating _____ out of seven lunches

My child is eating _____ out of seven dinners

Are they skipping snacks?

My child is eating _____ out of seven morning snacks

My child is eating _____ out of seven afternoon snacks

My child is eating _____ out of seven evening snacks

When your child eats, they use a:

Side salad or small plate

Large-size dinner plate

When your child eats, the plates are:

100 percent full

75 percent full

50 percent full

25 percent full

Name foods that your child consumes in each of the following categories:

_____

Grains/starches (examples: bread, rice, cereal, pasta)

_____

Proteins (examples: meat, poultry, fish, beans)

_____

Fruits

_____

Vegetables

_____

Fats (examples: butter, oil, avocado, nuts)

_____

Dairy (examples: milk, yogurt, cheese)

_____

Fluids (examples: water, milk, juice, coffee/tea)

_____

Snacks

Recall what your child's favorite meals used to be:

_____

Do you notice areas that are insufficient? If so, which areas need the most work?

Beginning Phase 1

As you learned in chapter 2, family-based treatment (FBT) includes three distinct phases. In Phase 1, you will be responsible for refeeding your child, taking over all aspects of the process while implementing the Plate-by-Plate approach. Phase 2 occurs once your child has shown some restoration of weight and health as well as compliance with implementation of the Plate-by-Plate approach. Gradually, activity and food independence will be added in leading up to Phase 3, where your child will regain food autonomy and some sense of normalcy returns.

Take Charge and Set Expectations

As the parent, you know best how to feed your child. Here in Phase 1 of FBT, parents are responsible for supervising all of their child's meals. You will take over all aspects of your child's food intake: grocery shopping, menu planning, meal preparation, and plating of meals.

Grocery shopping is something you should do *without* your child. Often, when accompanying parents, the child's eating disorder starts "talking" and will try to convince them to buy diet food: "triple-zero yogurt," "70-calorie bread," or "sugar-free oatmeal." You alone should make all food purchases until your child's eating disorder is much quieter and your child is in a stable enough place to be involved again. We recommend that foods purchased for your child be full fat, full sugar, and full carb, and that sugar-free foods, light foods, or fat-free items be avoided.

In the same way, a child with an eating disorder will often want to watch over their parents as they prepare meals, offering up suggestions or preferences. "Use less oil." "Don't add the sugar." "I will only eat the broccoli if it is steamed." "Preferences and suggestions" are usually in alignment with feeding your child's eating disorder rather than fighting it. Giving in to these demands perpetuates the fear associated with using oil, adding sugar, or adding sauce to foods. Your child should not be allowed in the kitchen at all during meal preparation.

Even though this book provides guidelines and suggestions for meals, you as the parent ultimately have the final say. If the meal looks too small, then you should add more food to the plate. If the meal feels too "diety," then you should adjust it to look more balanced. *This will need to happen despite protests from your child's eating disorder.*

Conversation with your child on the topic of food allows for the eating disorder to keep breathing. If you allow your child to have rice instead of bread because they insist it's "healthier," your child will remain fearful of bread. Your child's negotiations are a way to protect the eating disorder— to make the situation more tolerable for *the eating disorder*. And while agreeing with your child would be *so much easier*, we want you to make the decision that is most aligned with fighting your child's eating disorder, not the one that is easiest. You can, however, decide to serve an "easier meal" one night, but that decision has to come from you, not your child.

To be successful, you will need to set the expectation that your child *will* eat. This may take some practice in shifting how you think. "I wonder if she will like this pasta?" can be converted to "She will eat this pasta, whether she enjoys it or not." Similarly, "I know she won't eat this" becomes "She will eat everything on her plate, and we will support her through it." The commitment to recovery, to your child finishing their plate, to remaining steadfast in the fight against your child's eating disorder, is how you take back the table.

You should also avoid asking your child what they want for dinner. If you ask your child, "Do you want to try the pasta tonight?" Most kids with eating disorders will say no. Instead, you might say, "Tonight we will have pasta," or you can just serve the pasta, without encouraging a discussion about it.

You should plan to sit next to your child at all meals, and gently coach them as needed throughout the meal. Remind your child that they can do this, that you are here to help them, that you will fight the eating disorder and that you love them too much to let the eating disorder win. Try to talk about other things, which might be hard because you might feel anxious, and try to keep the conversation light and breezy. Talk about your day, or play games, as discussed later in this chapter. Games can be a great distraction. And then every so often as needed if your child zones out, remind them to pick up their fork, and take a bite.

What If My Child Won't Finish Eating?

At this stage, finishing what's on the plate should be prioritized above everything else, including school. Kids usually don't like missing school, or missing out on activities, but they will learn that their health is now a priority. That said, if the meal is dragging on, and you feel ready to move on, you can choose to use a supplement to ensure that your child gets in enough calories and doesn't fall behind on their meals. We recommend using a product like Ensure Plus or BOOST Plus (about 360 calories in an eight-ounce drink) to replace whatever is left on the plate. These products can be name brand or generic and can be found in most grocery stores and pharmacies as well as online.

Unfinished meals should be replaced with Ensure Plus– / BOOST Plus–type supplement within an hour from the time you started that meal to avoid running into the next meal or snack. You should feel free to use your judgment on this one. If a meal could have been completed in thirty minutes, allow thirty minutes for your child to complete it before requiring replacement with Ensure Plus/BOOST Plus. If you would expect your child to complete a snack within fifteen minutes, provide the replacement after that time is up.

Supplementing Protocol

Meals = two bottles

Snacks = one bottle

- If less than 50 percent of a meal is eaten, we recommend supplementing it with two bottles of Ensure Plus/BOOST Plus.
- If more than 50 percent of a meal is eaten, but not fully finished, we recommend supplementing it with one bottle of Ensure Plus/BOOST Plus.
- If less than 50 percent of a snack is eaten, we recommend supplementing with one bottle of Ensure Plus/BOOST Plus.
- If more than 50 percent of a snack is eaten, but not fully finished, we recommend supplementing with half a bottle of Ensure Plus/BOOST Plus.

What If My Child Gets Angry?

In order to truly fight the eating disorder, you will need to win, and win often. Each victory quiets the eating disorder. Each time your child eats your spaghetti, they are inching closer to freedom from their eating disorder.

Warning: this fight can get ugly. Plates may fly; your child may hit you, bite you, or throw your brand-new iPhone across the room. These behaviors, while not at all typical of your child before the eating disorder, are what we see when that monster of a disease is holding your child captive with its unrelenting grip. When your child's emotions escalate, you have hit a nerve. Don't back down in the face of this distress. Envision yourself as ripping the eating disorder from your child, fighting the eating disorder, and not allowing the eating disorder to "take" your child. The eating disorder can be fierce, and it will take united, strong, and empowered parents to defeat this beast.

Allow your child the space to be safely upset about the change in mealtime dynamics. Remember that your child is relinquishing complete control over their food choices and doing so involuntarily. They *will* be upset, and that's okay. What's not okay is for them to make you or anyone else in the family feel unsafe. Despite the tears and tantrums, expect your child to arrive at the table for all scheduled meals and snacks. If they refuse, make sure there is a direct consequence, e.g., they can no longer go to the mall with their friends that day because they didn't eat any food. If they aren't eating, they do not have the energy to walk around a mall with their friends.

If breakfast takes too long, then they might be late, or even need to miss school that day. Their health takes priority. Your child will quickly learn that you will not negotiate with the eating disorder and that meals are prioritized above all else. They will see that the fastest way to get their life and independence back is to prove they can take care of themselves by eating.

Nan Shaw, LCSW and family-based treatment expert (who wrote chapter 2), suggests that when your child throws food or yells, the FBT approach is to:

- Take a breath. Think, "The eating disorder is having a tantrum."
- Do your best to remain calm (and if you can't, ask another caregiver to take this lap).

The Plate-by-Plate Approach

- Remind yourself "This is the illness talking."
- Let your child know that you love them too much to let them hurt themselves, that you are in this fight against the eating disorder with them, and you will not give up on them.

If they throw the sandwich, simply make another one. If they are breaking cups or plates, use plastic ones. If they are hiding food, look in their rooms or the trash and determine what items got missed and replace those, and make sure your child has 100 percent supervision during all meals and snacks. If they beg you to stop insisting they complete a meal, know that they need the full dose of "medicine," even if it's challenging.

If you suspect purging, disallow the use of the bathroom for one hour after eating or insist they keep the door cracked open and sing a song or count out loud while in there. If they need to complete a meal with a supplement, that's still success, not failure. If they try to tamper with the lunch you prepared for them, make it inaccessible (one parent locked the lunch in a cooler in the trunk of her car every morning). If they run out of the house, expect them to eat when they come back and add in items for the running. And of course, if you are ever worried about your child's or your own safety, call 911.

Watch Closely

As your child progresses through the phases of FBT, the level of parental supervision will shift from watching every meal (Phase 1) to trusting that your child can get in all of their meals on their own (Phase 3). Phase 1 of FBT dictates that all meals should be supervised 100 percent. This includes lunch, even when your child is at school. Many parents will meet their child for lunch, or arrange for their child to be supervised by a teacher or the school nurse. Close and consistent supervision helps to fight the eating disorder while maximizing weight gain and nutritional rehabilitation.

During this process, it is imperative that parents supervise their child closely at mealtime. A child recovering from an eating disorder will look for any opportunity to minimize how much they have to eat during a meal. At this stage, they are often reluctant, or downright angry, about having to eat "this much." The eating disorder is manipulative and causes what was once a trustworthy reliable child to become sneaky, requiring supervision around meals at all times. We have caught kids hiding food in their boots or their napkin. We have seen sandwiches make their way into bras, pants, and socks if a parent isn't watching. Pay close attention to where the family dog is during meals. Dogs shouldn't be allowed near the table.

Nan Shaw says, "Try not to watch them like a hawk; instead think of it as if you are watching as a guardian angel." A firm but loving stance is most successful. Excessive focus, like a hawk, increases the stress and intensity at meals, making it more difficult for your child to eat. But if you see your child engaging in eating-disorder behaviors, such as letting food spill on their shirt or on the floor, redirect them, and make sure they know they need to stop that behavior. Try not to get upset, though we know that's easier said than done. The eating disorder has taken over your child's mind and body, causing them to act differently than ever before. At mealtimes, you should watch out for the following behaviors as previously described on page 24:

- Cutting food into extremely small pieces
- Ripping/pulling foods apart
- Excessive intake of fluids with meals/snacks
- Eating rapidly
- Organizing food on the plate before eating
- Eating foods in a specific order
- Letting food drop/spill on the floor or table, spilling beverages
- Hiding food (under dishes, napkins)
- Spitting food into napkins
- Excessive use of napkins/wiping mouth, hands, or silverware excessively
- Constant talking about food during the meal
- Eating slowly/taking small bites

Mealtime Talk

It can be helpful to brainstorm with your child and other family members what conversation topics are positive to talk about and which ones to avoid. This helps the home become a place of serenity in the face of an eating disorder—a safe zone, protected from the messages your child and your family are inundated with in the outside world. This will also give your family a chance to talk about other things: politics, sports, school, and friends! For that reason, it can be helpful for you and your family to decide on ground rules for family-time conversation.

SAFE TOPICS TO TALK ABOUT	CONVERSATION TOPICS TO AVOID
Politics	Anything about weight
School	Anything about dieting
Friends	Anything about cutting out foods or "good foods" or "bad foods"
Work	Other people's weight or shape
Family vacations	Your own health issues or concerns
Goals, dreams	Threatening your child to eat (this will only increase anxiety)

Mealtime is typically chaotic and stressful for a child with an eating disorder, so it is especially important to avoid talking about weight, shape, and body image during meals. Again, such comments create tension and stress, and remind your child about their desire to want to lose weight and eat less.

Positive food talk, such as saying how yummy something tastes, is generally safe to say and models "normal" eating. However, negative food talk should be discouraged at the table and beyond. Remarking on how "fatty the steak is" will only make the meal harder for your child. Other seemingly harmless comments like "Oh, I'm so full!" or "That dessert looks delicious, but I really shouldn't" need to be avoided entirely. It is helpful to imagine how your words will fall onto your child's ears. And if there is a question about whether they can hear what you're about to say, don't say it. Again, silence is golden here.

The following is an example of dining room rules created by teens at the Healthy Teen Project, an eating-disorder treatment program in Los Altos, California. The rules were created by the teens in order to make mealtime more peaceful. The list starts off setting the ground rules for the timing of meals: thirty minutes for a meal and fifteen minutes for a snack. The group asks everyone to "keep the environment and the conversation positive," refrain from using explicit language, don't talk about your body, include the whole community in the conversation, allow anyone in the group to "change the conversation at any time," and avoid all "discussion of portion sizes, meal plans, numbers, nutritional values, and activities."

Table Guidelines

You have 30 minutes for meals and 15 minutes for snack.

keep enviroment and conversation positive and supportive

Try to include entire community in conversation

No explict language. Keep it appropriate.

Refrain from discussing past treatment and/or hospital visits

Avoid discussion of portion sizes, meal plans, numbers, nutritional values, and activities

Avoid body image related talk

No negative food talk

Everyone has the right to change conversation topic at any time

Sleeves Rolled up, No big jackets, or Pockets

One Napkin, keep it Flat

One straw per day, only in water

Stay seated at the table, ask staff if you need something

July 2017

Mealtimes work best when there is fun, light conversation. Playing a game at the table can be a great way to distract your child from the stress associated with eating. Here is a list of great table games/conversation starters to keep mealtimes light and enjoyable. Families that have gone through this have found these games to be incredibly helpful for changing the tone at the table.

Fun Table-Game Ideas[1]

- **Twenty Questions:** One person thinks of something. The group then can ask twenty different questions to try to figure it out. "Is it a person, place, or thing?" or "Is it bigger than a building?" This can be a fun way to remember memories, and can really make you think—serving as a great distraction for any distress at the table.

- **Story Starters:** The group writes different words on small pieces of paper and places them in a bowl in the middle of the table. Each person at the table then chooses a word from the bowl. These words are now your "story starters." Using these words, the group tries to create a story.

- **20 Things I Love About . . .:** This is a great way to be positive, to increase gratitude and appreciation. The group can come up with a topic together, such as *winter* or my *teachers* or *Japan*. Each person is then asked to name something they love about that topic chosen, until you have twenty items. It is fun to take notes on this, which could be tricky while eating, and look back at it years later.

- **Would You Rather . . . ?:** It's fun to ask each other questions starting with "Would you rather . . . ?" These can get ridiculous and silly, and can be a great way to get to know your tablemates even better. Some examples include:
  - . . . own your own boat or your own plane?
  - . . . be able to fly or be invisible?
  - . . . speak every language in the world or play every instrument?
  - . . . live in the future or in the past?
  - . . . be the best player on a losing team or the worst player on a winning team?
  - . . . live in the city or the country?

You can also purchase these games: Teen TableTopics, Mad Gab, or Hedbanz (there are several versions, including Disney and kids). For more information about fun table games, check out the Family Dinner Project website at https://thefamilydinnerproject.org/fun /dinner-games/, which describes several creative table games for all ages. Most are appropriate for your child during treatment for an eating disorder, though please be advised that any games asking your child to discuss food or use food terms at the table, even if seemingly benign, may not be appropriate at this time.

CHAPTER 7

The Plate-by-Plate Approach

Making Sure Your Child Gets Enough Food

THE **PLATE-BY-PLATE** APPROACH was uniquely created to work in tandem with FBT. It is a visual tool that parents can use to refeed their child without the risk of it contributing to eating-disorder beliefs and behaviors. It does not rely on counting calories or measuring and eventually serves as a gateway to normal eating. This section outlines the steps to successful implementation of the Plate-by-Plate approach.

Step 1: Choose a Ten-Inch Plate

The actual plate you use is critical in the Plate-by-Plate approach. Since this is a visual approach to serving enough food, it relies on a simple dinner-size plate as its backbone. This will be the only tool you will need to master this approach—no measuring cups or measuring spoons required! The plate size should be roughly ten inches wide. We ask that you do not use side salad plates, toddler plates, paper plates, or plastic plates, which are generally too small. The best plates are smooth, without ridges or inner circles that might confuse both you and your child when serving. If you were only to fill the "inner circle," the volume provided would be insufficient.

Below are examples of plate designs to avoid:

Families that use these "inner circle" plates, inevitably fill the plate only to the inner circle.

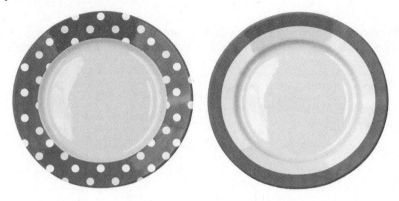

This is a better plate:

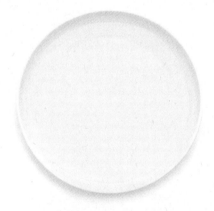

Step 2: Plate All Food Groups

The Plate-by-Plate approach will help you plate balanced meals. Each meal should include all five food groups: (1) grains/starches, (2) protein, (3) vegetables or fruits, (4) fats, and (5) dairy. What does this look like? Let's say you are making salmon for dinner. That covers the protein. What will your starch be? Potatoes? Sweet potatoes? Perhaps white rice sounds good? A salad could be your vegetable that night, and salad dressing could be the fat. Add a cup of milk, and all food groups are represented.

Food group checklist

A checklist like the following can be helpful in thinking about meal preparation and food purchasing to ensure that all food groups are represented during a meal.

FOOD GROUP	FOOD ITEM AT MEAL
GRAINS/STARCHES	
PROTEIN	
VEGETABLE OR FRUIT	
FAT	
DAIRY	

If all food groups are accounted for, the next step is to plate those food groups according to these criteria: 50 percent grains/starches, 25 percent protein, 25 percent fruits or vegetables, plus added fat and dairy. This means that grains/starches will visually take up half your child's dinner-size plate, with protein and fruits/vegetables making up the remaining quarters.

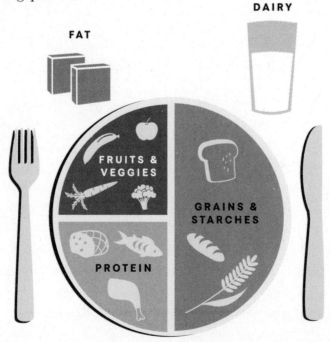

The Plate-by-Plate Approach

Food should be prepared with fats, and each meal should include dairy. Resist the urge to count calories or measure portions beyond this. If your child observes you doing that, or hears you talking that way about their plate, they will think that way, too.

In the next chapter, we will discuss why this breakdown of food groups best supports your child's recovery, and we will discuss what snacks look like and provide sample breakfasts, lunches, dinners, and snacks in chapter 9.

Step 3: Fill Up the Plate!

Now that you are clear on how big the plate should be and on the proportion of food groups recommended, the next step is to make sure it is "enough." *There should be no empty space left on the plate.* If you plate a meal and it covers only 60 percent or 75 percent of the plate, your portions are too small. You may think you are following the Plate-by-Plate approach because the plate contains all the food groups, but a sparse plate is an incomplete plate. The meal pictured below shows a plate that has protein (chicken), fruit/vegetables (string beans), grains/starch (mashed potatoes), fat (butter in the mashed potatoes), and dairy (glass of milk, not pictured)—but the plate isn't full.

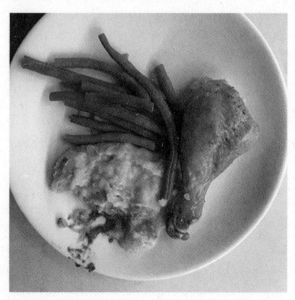

We liken this increase to "ripping off the Band-Aid." Many years ago, parents were taught to increase the volume of their child's plate slowly. Newer research shows that it is safe to jump to more calorically dense meals and an overall higher caloric meal plan right away.[1] We suggest parents jump right to the full plate, rather than starting with less and working their way up. A more rapid recovery is associated with a more favorable prognosis.[2] Given the relative safety of increasing the volume of food consumed, the faster your child becomes weight-restored, the better the long-term outcome.

That said, if your child does not have a lot of weight to gain, or if you feel certain your child would be more psychologically distressed with such a drastic change in the meal plan (note: most kids will have psychological distress during this time), you can proceed more slowly. But we have often found that these kids are more likely to remain sick, struggling more to progress with their meals.

A completely full plate may feel like a lot of food to you. The volume required during this process will be high, often higher than parents can imagine; the volume of food might be roughly twice what the child's mother eats and 1.5 times what her father eats. Therefore, it doesn't help to compare what your child eats to what you eat; they should be eating *way* more than you!

Remember, adolescence is a time of rapid growth and development, requiring increased caloric demands anyway. Gender, body size, growth rate, and activity level specifically determine how many calories teens need. Healthy teenage boys on average need 1,800 to 2,600 calories a day if they're eleven to thirteen years old, and 2,200 to 3,200 calories a day if they're fourteen to eighteen years of age. Healthy teenage girls need more, too: 1,800 to 2,200 calories a day if they're ages eleven to thirteen, and 1,800 to 2,400 calories a day if they're ages fourteen to eighteen. Those involved in strenuous physical activity such as soccer, basketball, football, or other sports may need even more calories to meet their nutritional needs.[3] If your child is an athlete, additional calories may be required. For example, if your child is running track, they may need an additional 400 to 500 calories (or more!) per day on top of their baseline requirement to support weight gain. A teenager with an eating disorder will require even more than this if weight gain is indicated as part of their treatment goals.

The volume of food required to keep gaining weight will increase as your child's metabolism increases, making it harder to restore weight. We will discuss how to continue to increase the caloric density and volume of the plates during the later stages of refeeding in chapter 11.

Step 4: Decide How Many Meals; How Many Snacks

The initial goal is three meals plus two or three snacks per day. Whether your child should start with two snacks or three depends on how many snacks your child is currently having. If your child is having two snacks, but they are small, you can begin by increasing the size of the snack. If your child is already having two snacks that each include at least two or three items, then you can either make those snacks larger or add a third snack. Your dietitian can help guide you as to what is the best first goal.

Snacks should contain two to three food groups each to start (any food groups of your choice) and will increase as the meal plan increases. We ask that you do not use two of the same food groups in one snack in order to improve variety. Your child may say, "Okay, I will have an apple and banana for my two items." Remind your child that they need two unique food groups, such as yogurt (dairy) and pretzels (grain). Limit fruits and vegetables as snacks, as they are the least calorically dense of all food groups. Examples of good snack choices are provided in chapter 9.

Step 5: Include a Variety of Foods

Variety is an essential component to the Plate-by-Plate approach. It is important that your child has different breakfasts, lunches, dinners, and snacks. Your child may try to convince you that they "just love oatmeal so much" and "that's all (they) want to eat in the morning." If there were no eating disorder present, the lack of variety would be less concerning, since your child would likely be getting enough of a balance of foods throughout the day to grow and develop. However, a child with an eating disorder often gets stuck in the same pattern because they are scared to try something different. This fear may be due to the fact that they deem another choice to be unhealthy or too processed, or they are scared that "those types of foods" will make them fat. It is important to break that way of thinking as early as possible and to show them that having cold cereal or waffles instead of oatmeal will not make them fat. Most parents know this intuitively, but they are scared to fight against their child's fierce eating disorder (and rightfully so!). The eating disorder conditions parents to live in fear—it rears its ugly head at every meal when challenged, and only quiets when its food rules are accommodated. Insisting that your child change will disrupt the peace in your home and potentially lead to yelling and tears. It is *much easier* to give in and let your child eat the same thing every day, but that won't fight the eating disorder. The end goal is for your child to be truly free to eat anything, to be flexible and open to all foods. Kids whose food choices remain restrictive struggle to attend parties, social outings, and college. For more on variety and including all types of foods in your child's diet, see Chapter 14: Moving Beyond Brown Rice.

Step 6: Do a Final Review: How Does the Plate Look?

Use this last step as a final run-through of how the plate looks. Ask yourself: Does the plate make sense? Sure, it has all the food groups present, but do these foods go together? For example, avoid serving chicken with a side of cereal and milk, or salmon with pretzels. The meal should be cohesive and feel "normal." On the facing page is an example of a plate that does not make sense. One of our patients, further along in recovery, was working on becoming more independent with plating her own meals. In her most earnest attempt to follow the plate model and include all the food groups, she plated crab (protein) with manicotti pasta (dairy/starch/fats), snap peas (veggies), popcorn (to make sure she had enough starch), and a coconut protein beverage. In her best attempt to follow the guidelines, the meal ended up not making sense. We directed her to take out the crab, double the manicotti pasta (adds more grain and more protein), get rid of the popcorn, and add a dipping sauce for the snap peas (dressing, hummus, or guacamole adds fat), and substitute the coconut protein beverage for a glass of milk (adds dairy). These changes make a cohesive meal out of a random assortment of food while ensuring all food groups are present.

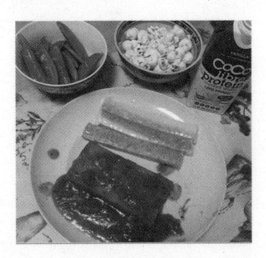

As you review your child's plate, ask yourself these questions:

- Are all food groups present? Grains/starches? Protein? Fruit or vegetable? Dairy? Fat?
- Is the plate 50 percent grains/starches, 25 percent protein, 25 percent fruit or vegetable?
- Is the whole plate full?
- Does the meal "make sense" and feel cohesive?
- Have you challenged your child?

CHAPTER 8

——◦—◦——

Why This Breakdown?

A Close-up on Grains/Starches, Proteins, Fruits and Vegetables, Fats, and Dairy

PARENTS ARE OFTEN inundated with food and health messages, and the recommendations for what their child needs can be easily blurred. *Are carbohydrates "bad?" Should my child eat more protein to gain muscle weight? Should they limit fats?* Yet an adolescent with an eating disorder has their own unique nutrition needs. This chapter explores what the recommendations are for carbohydrates, protein, dairy, fats, and fruits/vegetables as part of your child's recovery.

Grains and Starches: 50 Percent of the Plate

Carbohydrates, found in high concentrations in the grains/starches food group, unjustly have a bad reputation. People say things like carbs "make me bloated," "make me gain weight," or "make me tired." For every positive thing you have read about carbohydrates, you have most likely read something negative. As the United States struggles with an obesity epidemic, the health messaging to "cut back on carbs" or "reduce simple sugars" has been widespread and hard to ignore. Navigating what's healthy for a teen can be confusing, especially given all the messaging that is typically geared toward adults. Much of what you read in the media is based on pseudoscience, as well as people's reactions or feelings, and is not grounded in findings from well-designed studies.

The truth is, carbohydrates are one of three major macronutrients that the body needs (the others are protein and fat). When carbohydrates are digested, they are broken down into glucose. Glucose is carried through the blood to give energy to all parts of the body, including the brain, muscles, organs, and tissues.

Carbohydrates should cover half of your child's plate.[1] Now, this will likely be a shift from what your child is currently eating, or even from what your family is eating. But it's necessary to resolve the medical complications associated with eating disorders. The plate should be 50 percent grains/starches in order for your child's body to have enough energy to perform basic functions such as allowing their heart to pump blood efficiently, keeping their body warm, and for girls to maintain a monthly menstrual cycle. Anything less than that is likely to compromise the body's functioning.

Carbohydrate-rich foods include breads, wraps, rolls, bagels, cereals, oatmeal, couscous, quinoa, rice, potatoes, pizza, pasta, cookies, fries, pretzels, and granola bars, just to name a few. While creating a plate that is 50 percent grains/starches, you may certainly combine them. For example, you can serve a plate that is 25 percent quinoa and 25 percent rice. As long as the total plate looks to be 50 percent starch and feels cohesive, anything can work here.

Although fruit and milk technically contain carbohydrates (fruits contain fructose, and milk contains lactose), we do not count that toward the half a plate of grains. This helps to ensure that the volume and balance of food is sufficient to meet energy requirements. In fact, to fulfill the "grains/starches" portion of the plate, we look only to grains (rice, pasta, bread, etc.) and potatoes. While it is true that other starchy foods such as beans and corn may fit into this category, it is recommended to think of them as protein (beans) or vegetables (corn). This will help to keep the diet adequately balanced, providing enough calories while also minimizing gassiness or bloating associated with higher fiber content in starchy vegetables.

Provide a Variety of Grains

Kids with eating disorders tend to have a diet with limited variety. They will say, "I don't mind, I like brown rice." But often this limited diet is directly tied to their eating disorder. Kids may have arbitrarily eliminated gluten or decided they can only eat "whole grains." Their limited diet is often coming from a place of fear, and parents should feel empowered to work through this fear with their child to fully conquer the eating disorder. A rotation of grains/starches is important to make sure your child is getting an assortment of nutrients and exposure to several different types of food. Parents must strategize how best to incorporate other foods into their child's diet. The more variety parents provide, the less rigidity their child will have around food in the long run. Think back to when you were introducing new foods to your child when they were a baby. Similarly, rotating from rice to quinoa to potatoes to pasta will ensure that your child gets comfortable with all foods while benefiting from the most nutrients.

Certain grains/starches may be more palatable to your child. For example, your child might decide they only want quinoa. Some parents will feel relieved. "At least they eat." Eating *only* quinoa and *never* pasta or white rice, however, reinforces a food hierarchy, where your child views some foods as "better" or "healthier" than others. In order for your child to be free of the eating disorder, all foods must be allowed. We will discuss strategies for exposure in Chapter 14: Moving Beyond Brown Rice. The more variety you include, the better your child will be at navigating situations outside the home, such as parties, restaurants, and travel.

Proteins: 25 Percent of the Plate

In the United States, the average teenager's diet far exceeds the recommended daily allowance for protein, and teens are rarely deficient. However, with an eating disorder, the child's rules and restrictions may cause their diet to become out of balance. The Plate-by-Plate approach recommends that the plate be made up of 25 percent protein. This target amount, combined with the protein that will also come from dairy foods, will ensure that your child consumes an appropriate amount of protein throughout the day to support their growth and development. During refeeding, protein will be necessary for your child to regain muscle mass in their extremities (arms and legs) and in vital organs such as the heart, liver, kidneys, and lungs. Protein, in combination with carbohydrates, will help with the rebuilding process necessary to get your child healthy again.

Many popular diets today, such as Paleo, Atkins, and South Beach diets, are protein-focused, with carbohydrates being limited or excluded. Parents familiar with these diets may wonder if the plate being "only" 25 percent protein is enough—but trust us, it is! If you follow this structure, your child's protein intake will be more than adequate. For example, a four-ounce breast of chicken has around twenty-eight grams of protein and is an appropriate volume to make up 25 percent of the plate. A mildly active 115-pound girl, one who is not involved in strength training, requires only around fifty grams of protein *for the whole day* based on the recommended daily allowance of protein, which is a set 0.4 to 0.5 grams of protein per pound of body weight.[2] That means that with only one four-ounce breast of chicken (or 25 percent of the plate coming from protein), one plate would provide more than half of your child's protein needs for the day.

A diet skewed to contain a higher amount of protein is difficult for kids with eating disorders to tolerate. Protein has a high satiety factor and takes longer to leave the stomach. Because of this, a high-protein diet would make it more difficult for your child to follow the meal plan with consistency— meal after meal, snack after snack. With too much protein, you will hear complaints of "feeling too full" (we expect that to happen anyway during refeeding, but too much protein can intensify the feeling). We know this process may cause your child to be physically uncomfortable, but the goal is to minimize gastrointestinal distress, which occurs less often when the protein portion is set at 25 percent. Too much protein can also worsen constipation, which is likely to occur during the refeeding process.

We suggest a variety of proteins, such as chicken, turkey, fish, shellfish, beef, buffalo, bison meat, lamb, pork, eggs, beans, tofu, seitan (wheat gluten), or tempeh. Dairy sources can be used as a protein but cannot *also* count as your child's dairy source for that meal (you would need to count a yogurt as either the dairy or protein; it can't be both). We discuss this further as we cover the dairy section of the plate on page 136. Ideally, your child would be eating the same meals that your family is eating, without any substitutions.

Variety is important in order to broaden your child's palate and ensure that they are getting a wide range of nutrients. For example, if your child only eats chicken and fish, they will be missing out on the iron found in red meat. Iron is responsible for bringing oxygen to various parts of the body, giving them energy to perform. Low iron levels may cause your child to feel tired, weak, or irritable. If they are an athlete, this will be noticeable on the field and should be corrected. Female athletes are at greater risk for developing iron-deficiency than nonathletes, and female athletes who are vegetarian have an even higher likelihood of having low iron levels. If your child does not eat much red meat, is a vegetarian, and/or is an athlete, iron levels should be checked.

Dietary Sources of Iron

Iron can either come from meat sources or plant-based foods. Iron found in animal products is called heme iron, and iron found in plant-based foods is called non-heme iron. Heme iron is considered more biologically available, meaning it is better absorbed than plant-based iron and is found in highest quantities in liver, clams, oysters, and beef. For this reason, we suggest including red meat at least two to three times a week if that fits with your family's food beliefs.

Non-heme iron is found in beans, breakfast cereals, fortified bars, dark chocolate, raisins, and dark leafy greens (though the iron is harder to absorb in greens due to the presence of phytates). Plant sources of iron require a "vitamin C helper" in order for the body to completely absorb it. A list of vitamin C helpers follows and includes oranges, orange juices, cantaloupe, mango, red peppers, and tomatoes. A high consumption of tea and coffee inhibit iron absorption and should be limited.

Dietary Sources of Vitamin C

Add a Vitamin C Helper to Aid Iron Absorption

	SERVING SIZE	VITAMIN C (MG)
FRUIT/FRUIT JUICES		
Orange juice	1 cup	379
Grapefruit juice	1 cup	248
Peaches, frozen	1 cup	236
Oranges	1 cup	121
Mango	1 cup	60
Tangerine	1 cup	52
VEGETABLES/VEGETABLE JUICES		
Red peppers, chopped	1 cup	190
Tomato juice, canned	1 cup	170
Peppers, green	1 cup	120
Broccoli	1 cup	88
Peas	1 cup	58
Tomatoes	1 cup	30

What If My Child Is a Vegetarian?

We are seeing an increasing number of teens becoming vegetarian or vegan. A healthy vegetarian diet is certainly possible with careful planning, yet an eating disorder often creates several limitations that make meeting one's nutritional goals more challenging. Teens choose to become vegetarian for a variety of reasons. They may have watched a movie at school about animal rights, have a friend whose family is vegetarian, or they may have always been "picky" about meat. Often, we see kids become vegetarians just as their eating disorder is beginning. If your child is a vegetarian, when did they convert? How long were they a vegetarian before the eating disorder began? This timing is critical: the closer the start of the vegetarianism is to the onset of the eating disorder, the higher the likelihood that the vegetarianism is *part* of the eating disorder. If your child's vegetarianism is found to be intertwined with their eating disorder, then it is important to have your child eat meat. A common recommendation we make is that a child must be weight-restored, and for girls to have at least three consecutive periods, before we would consider letting a child resume vegetarian eating. At that point, it would be up to the child's treatment team to assess whether the timing is right and whether it makes sense based on where they are in their recovery.

There are some instances where vegetarianism can be permitted during recovery. But it is important to tease out whether your child is using the vegetarianism as a means of keeping their eating disorder alive. We work with plenty of kids who are vegetarians *and* have eating disorders. Vegetarianism is allowed when the child has been a vegetarian for far longer than they have had an eating disorder, or when the whole family is vegetarian. In these cases, a child would have our blessing to continue a vegetarian diet.

If your child is a vegetarian, the Plate-by-Plate approach can still be followed. Instead of meat-based proteins, 25 percent of the plate would come from eggs, beans, tofu, tempeh, nuts, seeds, and nut butters. Dairy can also be a good source of protein. We provide sample vegetarian meal plans in Chapter 9: Putting It All Together.

A note on veganism: given the low-caloric density of most plant-based foods and the high volume of roughage required to fill a vegan plate, it is not advised for a child with an eating disorder to follow a vegan diet. If your family is vegan, it may be worth considering allowing your child to eat a lacto-ovo (including dairy and eggs) vegetarian diet while undergoing treatment for their eating disorder. If this isn't possible, special attention should be paid to make sure a dairy equivalent is used that provides sufficient protein and calcium.

Finally, a multivitamin is recommended for all vegetarians/vegans whose diet may be lacking vitamin B12, a vitamin found only in animal products (and some fortified foods such as bars and some beverages), and iron (vegetarians have a higher daily requirement for iron).

Fruits and Vegetables: 25 Percent of the Plate

While fruits and vegetables are nutritious and an important component of your child's meals, we limit them to a quarter of the plate for several

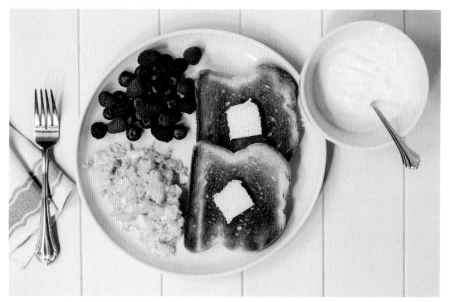

BREAKFAST PLATE: *Starch (50%), toast; Protein (25%), scrambled eggs; Fruit/ Veg (25%), mixed berries; Fat, butter; Dairy, yogurt*

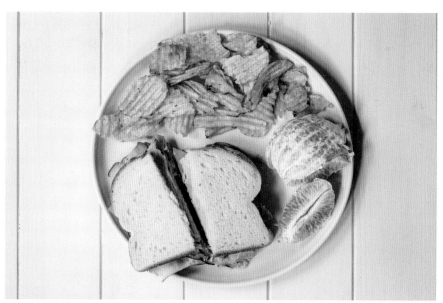

LUNCH PLATE: *Starch (50%), sandwich bread + chips; Protein (25%), turkey slices; Fruit/Veg (25%), orange; Fat, mayonnaise (in sandwich); Dairy, cheddar cheese (in sandwich)*

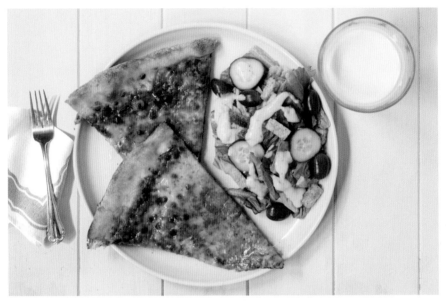

LUNCH PLATE: *Starch (50%), pizza crust; Protein (25%), cheese (on pizza); Fruit/Veg (25%), tossed salad; Fat, salad dressing; Dairy, glass of milk*

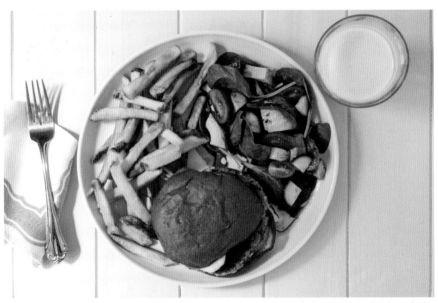

VEGETARIAN DINNER PLATE: *Starch (50%), bun + french fries; Protein (25%), veggie burger; Fruit/Veg (25%), tossed salad; Fat, avocado + salad dressing; Dairy, glass of milk*

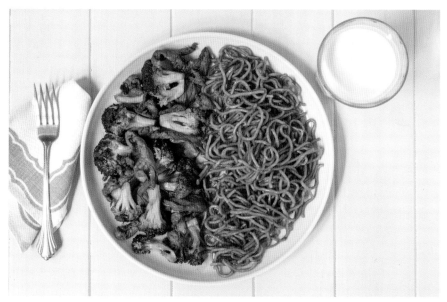

CHINESE DINNER PLATE: *Starch (50%), lo mein; Protein (25%), beef; Fruit/Veg (25%), broccoli; Fat, oil (for cooking lo mein and beef); Dairy, glass of milk*

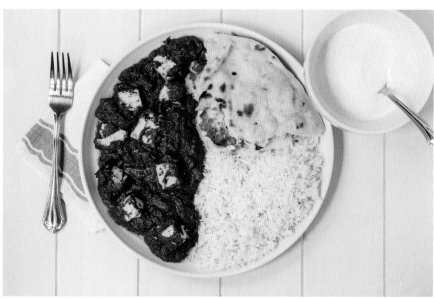

INDIAN DINNER PLATE: *Starch (50%), rice + ½ piece naan; Protein (25%), paneer (cheese in curry); Fruit/Veg (25%), spinach; Fat, ghee (in curry); Dairy, yogurt*

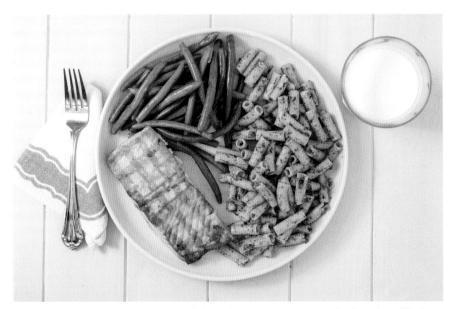

STANDARD DINNER PLATE: *Starch (50%), pesto pasta; Protein (25%), grilled salmon; Fruit/Veg (25%), sautéed green beans; Fat, oil (in pesto + on green beans); Dairy, glass of milk*

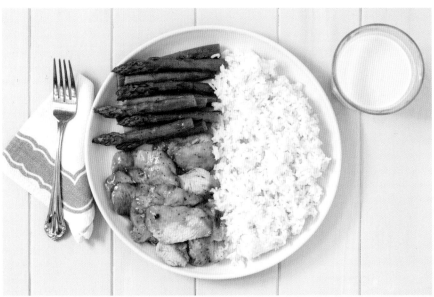

ACCELERATED PLATE: *Starch (heaping 50%), rice; Protein (25%), chicken teriyaki; Fruit/Veg (25%), asparagus; Fat, sauce (on chicken); Dairy (milk in shake), nutritional shake*

Note: For more ideas on increasing the caloric density of the plate see pages 152 to 154.

reasons. Adolescents with eating disorders often consume an excess of fruits and vegetables, such as "a whole bag of spinach" or "an entire head of cauliflower." Excessive fruit and vegetable consumption ultimately needs to be reduced to make room for more calorically dense foods that will help with weight gain. In addition, gastrointestinal distress is common during the refeeding process as the body and metabolism get acclimated to this new way of eating. Reducing fruits and vegetables can help minimize gas and abdominal distention (otherwise known as "bloating").

For parents of kids with eating disorders, getting a child to cut back on the volume of fruits and vegetables may be more difficult than getting them to consume these foods in the first place. Watch out for "pretty plates" that are colorful and look full but are missing the right breakdown of nutrients. This will result in your child feeling full, and possibly bloated/gassy, while not getting in enough calories overall.

If your child is eating a lot of fruits and vegetables, you might want to take a look at the palms of their hands and the bottoms of their feet. Are they tinted orange? Assuming your child has not been playing with self-tanner, this orange-tinted pigmentation might be hypercarotenemia, as discussed in chapter 4.

Hypercarotenemia can happen to anyone who consumes an excess of carotenoids (found in carrots, red peppers, sweet potatoes, and other fruits and vegetables), usually in the absence of a varied diet. Typically, a hypercarotenemic child is eating an excessive amount of fruits and vegetables while not consuming enough fats, carbohydrates, or protein. A high carotene level in and of itself is not dangerous, but is symbolic of your child's unbalanced diet. Your doctor can order a baseline carotene level and can track it throughout the nutritional rehabilitation process. As the child's diet improves, the carotene levels will decrease. You can track it yourself simply by watching your child become "less orange" as their nutrition improves. If you suspect your child has hypercarotenemia, we suggest you limit your child's consumption of high carotenoid foods (see chart).

Beta-Carotene Content of Selected Foods

FOOD	SERVING	BETA CAROTENE (MG)
Sweet potato, boiled	1 cup	31.0
Carrot juice	1 cup	22.0
Pumpkin, canned	1 cup	17.0
Collards, cooked	1 cup	11.6
Kale, chopped	1 cup	11.5
Spinach, cooked	1 cup	11.3
Carrots, raw	1 cup, chopped	10.6
Winter squash, baked	1 cup	7.3
Cantaloupe, raw	1 cup	3.6
Apricots, dried	1 cup, halves	2.8
Peppers, sweet, red	1 cup, chopped	2.4
Mango, raw	1 cup	1.1

Fats

Consuming enough fats is often a struggle for those with eating disorders. Perhaps the word *fat* feels scary; they fear that "fats will make them fat." But no one food has the power to cause weight gain. Weight gain results when a person's caloric intake exceeds their caloric requirements. Eating above that caloric threshold will result in weight gain, regardless of whether the "extra" comes from apples or turkey or chocolate. All people of all ages require fats in their diet, regardless of their weight goals.

Eating fats has many advantages during the nutritional rehabilitation process. One of the most important attributes of fats is that they are an essential precursor for estrogen and testosterone synthesis. Dietary fats can actually help boost estrogen levels (in girls), which helps achieve menstruation and improve bone density, and testosterone levels (in boys) to promote growth, strength, and improved bone density. Adding back fats (and calories) is an essential part of correcting these hormonal imbalances. For those female teens who are weight-restored and still not getting a period, the diet may provide some answers as to how to boost hormone levels. Adding fats of any kind, whether avocado, nuts, salmon, chocolate, or cookies, can help restore hormone levels to normal.

Fats also help the body absorb the fat-soluble vitamins A, D, E, and K. Without enough dietary fat, these vitamins cannot be absorbed.

Vitamins That Require Fat for Absorption

Here is a quick snapshot on what these vitamins do for the body and why they are needed:

Vitamin A

- Necessary for vision, bone growth, and reproduction
- Involved in gene expression, affects the role of every cell in the body
- Plays a role in regulating the immune system and fighting infection

Vitamin D

- Necessary to absorb calcium and important for bone health
- Associated with immune function and may serve to protect against certain cancers

Vitamin E

- A powerful antioxidant necessary for protecting the cells from damage caused by free radicals, which can come from the food we eat or from the environment
- Helps to keep the immune system strong against viruses and bacteria
- Important in the formation of red blood cells and in the body's use of vitamin K; also helps widen blood vessels and keep blood from clotting inside them

Vitamin K

- Necessary for blood coagulation (clotting), bone metabolism, prevention of vessel mineralization, and regulation of various cellular functions

All meals and all snacks should contain fats. We suggest avoiding light or diet foods and choosing dairy products that are 2 percent fat or greater. Stay away from fat-free, 0 percent, light, or triple-zero yogurt. Here are more strategies for boosting the fat content of all meals.

Strategies for Getting More Fat on Your Child's Plate

Breakfast

- Spread a nut butter like peanut butter or almond butter on toast, an English muffin, or a bagel. Or mix a nut butter into oatmeal or add it to a smoothie.
- Sprinkle nuts on top of full-fat granola or mix them into oatmeal.
- Spread butter on toast, English muffins, or a bagel.
- Add avocado or guacamole to toast or breakfast burritos.

Lunch

- Use mayo on sandwiches.
- Add avocado or guacamole to sandwiches.
- Add hummus to sandwiches or on the side as a dip.
- Dip veggies in ranch dressing.
- Add a side that contains fat, such as a cookie, chocolate, trail mix, nuts, or chips.
- Add cheese (Note: can be counted as fats if not already used as a dairy, otherwise add an additional serving).
- Add seeds such as sunflower seeds, pumpkin seeds, or hemp seeds.

Dinner

- Add additional oil *after* cooking (30 percent evaporates during the cooking process).
- Add butter or oil to bread, pasta, rice, or veggies.
- Add chips as a side.
- Cook with sauces that contain fat (for example, a cream sauce or cheese sauce).

- Use salad dressing. (Salad should never be dry!)
- Sprinkle nuts, such as candied pecans or walnuts, and seeds onto salads.
- Add feta or goat cheese to a salad or sprinkle on top of veggies.
- Add avocado to a salad.

Dairy

Adolescence is a unique period of life during which a person can still add to their bone density. Accruing as much bone density as possible during adolescence is essential for optimizing bone health later in life. Dairy is an important food group for all adolescents, with and without eating disorders. If an eating disorder is present, a person's bones may be more at risk for having reduced bone density.

Calcium is needed to build strong bones and is highest in dairy products. Adequate vitamin D levels are necessary to absorb calcium. Having a diet that provides enough dietary fat is essential for absorbing vitamin D. Without enough fat in your child's diet, they won't be able to utilize calcium because their body won't be able to absorb it. This is why getting higher-fat milk is important. Whole and 2 percent milk have fat, vitamin D, and calcium, all of which immediately maximize calcium utilization.

The Plate-by-Plate approach includes a dairy source at each meal. The recommended daily allowance for teen boys and girls is 1,300 milligrams of calcium per day, which works out to roughly four servings of dairy per day.[3] Dairy sources include a glass of milk, yogurt, cottage cheese, kefir probiotic drink, and full-fat cheese. If your child likes cheese sticks, which are easy to pack in lunches, pack two, as they are lower in fat and calories than regular cheese.

Some people are lactose intolerant or intolerant to dairy. If this is the case for your child, we suggest using lactase enzymes (available over the counter) with the first bite of a dairy food or lactose-free milk when possible. If your child still can't tolerate milk or never liked it (which we hear a lot), you can consider a dairy-free alternative. Soy milk is your best bet, as it is usually fortified with calcium and vitamin D, contains fat (assuming it's not a fat-free variety), and has the same amount of protein as cow's milk per cup. Other nondairy milks such as almond milk, cashew milk, and rice milk have a different nutrient profile from dairy milk. Almond milk tends to be most popular with eating disorders because it is low in calories (forty-five per cup), low in fat, and low in protein. Therefore, we prefer to call almond "milk" almond "beverage" and recommend against using it for the nutritional rehabilitation process.

Lastly, because milk is so high in protein (eight grams per cup), it can sometimes be used as your child's protein source. But please note: dairy cannot serve as both your child's protein and dairy source; one food cannot count as two food groups. In this case, if your child is using milk as both dairy and protein at breakfast, then they would need two servings or a very tall glass: one serving would count as dairy and the other would count as protein.

Strategies for Getting More Dairy on Your Child's Plate

Breakfast
- Add a glass of milk to drink or to use in cereal.
- Prepare oatmeal with milk instead of water.
- Include yogurt or cottage cheese.
- Serve kefir, a probiotic smoothie drink, on the side.
- Add cheese to scrambled eggs.
- Add portable cheese sticks or Babybel cheese on the side (remember to serve two, as these are lower-calorie cheese options).
- Make a fruit smoothie with milk or yogurt.

Lunch
- Add a glass of milk or chocolate milk to drink. Look for shelf-stable or individual-size boxes that don't require refrigeration and can be packed for school lunches easily.
- Add cheese to sandwiches.
- Serve yogurt or kefir on the side.
- Crumble feta cheese or goat cheese over a salad.
- Use a spreadable cheese like Brie on sandwiches.

Dinner

- Add a glass of milk or chocolate milk to drink.
- Add yogurt or kefir on the side.
- Top a stir-fry or cooked broccoli with shredded cheese.
- Add Parmesan cheese to pasta dishes.
- Melt cheese on bread or in a quesadilla.
- Crumble blue cheese or goat cheese over a salad.
- Add ice cream at the end of the meal.

Common Foods by Food Group

GRAINS/ STARCHES	PROTEINS	FRUITS AND VEGETABLES	DAIRY	FATS
Bread	Beans	Apples	Buttermilk	Avocado
Cereal	Chicken	Asparagus	Cheese	Butter
Corn	Halibut	Bananas	Cottage cheese	Cream cheese
Couscous	Ham	Blackberries	Kefir	Guacamole
French fries	Hamburger	Blueberries	Milk, 2 percent	Hummus
French toast	Meatballs	Bok choy	Milk, Lactaid	Mayo
Oatmeal	Nut butters	Broccoli	Milk, whole	Nut butters
Pancakes	(peanut, almond,	Grapes	Milk, soy	(peanut, almond,
Pasta, white	cashew, etc.)	Juice	Paneer	cashew, etc.)
Pasta, wheat	Roast beef	Kale	Smoothie with	Nuts
Pita	Salmon	Mushrooms	milk	Oil
Pizza	Seitan	Nectarines	Tzatziki	Salad dressing
Potatoes	Shrimp	Oranges	Yogurt	Seeds
Quinoa	Steak	Plums		Sour cream
Rice, white	Swordfish	Salad		Whipped cream
Rice, brown	Tempeh	Strawberries		
Rice, yellow	Tilapia	Spinach		
Rolls	Tofu	Swiss chard		
Sweet potatoes	Turkey			
Waffles				
Wraps				

CHAPTER 9

Putting It All Together

Meal and Snack Ideas

THIS CHAPTER IS dedicated to putting the plate together and to making sure you have an idea of what a healthy plate for refeeding your child looks like. We will provide examples of how to critically assess each plate you provide, and will go through plate examples of good plates, and not-so-good plates. You'll be a pro at this in no time!

Plate-by-Plate: Breakfast

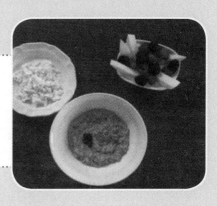

FOOD GROUP CHECKLIST

GRAINS/STARCHES	Fruit salad
PROTEIN	Oatmeal
VEGETABLES OR FRUIT	Egg
FAT	Nuts, but very little
DAIRY	Yogurt under fruit

FINAL REVIEW QUESTIONS

Are all food groups present? Grains/starches? Protein? Fruit/Veggies? Dairy? Fat?

✓ YES

Is the plate 50 percent grains/starches, 25 percent protein, 25 percent fruit/veggies?

✗ NO, this is one serving of oatmeal. It does not equate to 50 percent grains/starches.

Is the whole plate full?

✗ NO, there's too little grains/starches, too little fat.

Does the meal "make sense" and feel cohesive?

✓ YES

Have you challenged your child?

This looks like a "safe" breakfast. Aim to expand on variety and amount.

RECOMMENDATIONS

- Increase grains/starches (add more oatmeal or add toast).
- Increase fats (add more nuts or add butter to the oatmeal).
- Work on serving more challenging foods.

For additional examples of good plates see photo insert.

Plate-by-Plate: Lunch

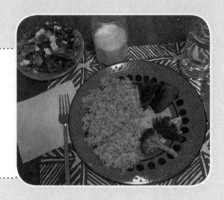

GRAINS/STARCHES	Brown rice
PROTEIN	Steak
VEGETABLES OR FRUIT	Broccoli, side salad
FAT	Dressing on salad
DAIRY	Feta cheese on salad, milk

FINAL REVIEW QUESTIONS

Are all food groups present? Grains/starches? Protein? Fruit/Veggies? Dairy? Fat?

✓ YES

Is the plate 50 percent grains/starches, 25 percent protein, 25 percent fruits/veggies?

✗ NO, there's not enough meat.

Is the whole plate full?

✗ NO. The meal is plated using the "inner circle," so overall it looks a bit light.

Does the meal "make sense" and feel cohesive?

✓ YES

Have you challenged your child?

✓ YES and **✗ NO**. Steak is challenging, so serving it here is great. Rotate grains to challenge variety (white rice, potatoes, etc.).

RECOMMENDATIONS

- For now, add more meat on the plate.
- Increase grain variety, as brown rice is often considered a "safe" food and does not challenge the "food rules" of a child with an eating disorder.
- Plate the food over the whole plate, and avoid using the inner circle as a guide.

For additional examples of good plates see photo insert.

The Plate-by-Plate Approach

Plate-by-Plate: Dinner

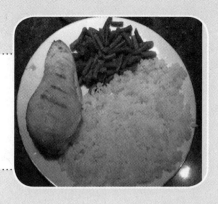

FOOD GROUP CHECKLIST

GRAINS/STARCHES	White rice
PROTEIN	Chicken
VEGETABLES OR FRUIT	Green beans
FAT	None
DAIRY	None

FINAL REVIEW QUESTIONS

Are all food groups present? Grains/starches? Protein? Fruit/Veggies? Dairy? Fat?

✗ NO, dairy and fats are missing.

Is the plate 50 percent grains/starches, 25 percent protein, 25 percent fruits/veggies?

✓ YES

Is the whole plate full?

✓ YES, excellent job here on that.

Does the meal "make sense" and feel cohesive?

✓ YES

Have you challenged your child?

✗ NO. This meal is a "safe" meal: plain grilled chicken, rice, and green beans are foods that this child is comfortable with already. And it looks very dry!

RECOMMENDATIONS

- For now, add dairy, such as a glass of milk.
- And add a fat, such as olive oil (visible to the eye) to the green beans or butter on the rice.
- Work on increasing variety of challenging foods.

For additional examples of good plates see photo insert.

Vegetarian Plate

Note: If your family is vegan and prefers your child remain vegan during treatment, soy products can be used in place of dairy. However, it is strongly recommended that you consider allowing your child to be lacto-ovo vegetarian during nutritional rehabilitation.

FOOD GROUP CHECKLIST

GRAINS/STARCHES	Saffron rice
PROTEIN	Kidney beans
VEGETABLES OR FRUIT	Cauliflower and snap peas
FAT	None
DAIRY	None

FINAL REVIEW QUESTIONS

Are all food groups present? Grains/starches? Protein? Fruit/Veggies? Dairy? Fat?

✗ NO, dairy and fats are missing.

Is the plate 50 percent grains/starches, 25 percent protein, 25 percent fruits/veggies?

✓ YES

Is the whole plate full?

✓ YES

Does the meal "make sense" and feel cohesive?

✓ YES

Have you challenged your child?

There is oil in the rice, and typically my child only eats brown rice, so this is a stretch.

RECOMMENDATIONS

- Add yogurt to fulfill the dairy group.
- Add hummus as a dip for the veggies.

For additional examples of good plates see photo insert.

Plate-by-Plate Snacks

Initially, we recommend you start with two snacks a day that include two items each. An "item" refers to a food item from one of the five food groups, and is equal to a typical serving of that food. For example, one serving of pretzels or one serving of nuts. (You can find these serving quantities on the package, but it's preferable for you to make your best guess on serving size to support your child's recovery and to normalize eating.) Good examples of a two-item snack would be yogurt and granola, or an apple and peanut butter.

It is important not to double up on food groups. Your child may ask for the snack to be a banana and raspberries, but we suggest you increase variety by offering foods from two different groups. We also suggest that you do not choose fruits and vegetables for both items, as the snack will not be nutritionally adequate. For example, a snack of carrots and blueberries is not a calorically dense snack and would not be appropriate for a child with an eating disorder. If you give your child an item that is more calorically dense, such as an energy bar, you may choose to pair it with a lighter item like fruit to balance it out. However, it is perfectly okay to serve some snacks that are more calorically dense than others—this will teach your child to be flexible and adaptable.

If your child is already eating two snacks and needs further weight gain, it may be time to increase either the number of snacks or the number of food items at each snack. If you choose to add a third item to your child's snacks, they will be similar to the following: apple and peanut butter and milk, or yogurt and granola and berries. An eight-ounce glass of juice serves as one item whereas a sixteen-ounce serving is two items. Many adolescents need three snacks per day to increase their overall intake, and this is a normal increase given their high energy demands.

Snacks can be increased as follows:

Two snacks, two items each

Example

Afternoon snack: apple and peanut butter

Evening snack: chocolate and banana

Two snacks, three items each

Example

Afternoon snack: apple, peanut butter, and milk

Evening snack: chocolate, banana, and yogurt

Three snacks, three items each

Example

Morning snack: energy bar (such as Nature Valley, KIND, or home-made), grapes, and eight ounces of juice

Afternoon snack: apple, peanut butter, and milk

Evening snack: chocolate, banana, and yogurt

Three snacks, four items each

Example

Morning snack: energy bar (such as Nature Valley, KIND, or home-made), grapes, and sixteen ounces of juice

Afternoon snack: apple, peanut butter—two servings (two items), and milk

Evening snack: chocolate—two servings (two items), banana, and yogurt

Here are more ideas for creating snacks.

Two-Item Snacks

- Apple and peanut butter
- Nuts and dried fruit
- Energy bar and grapes
- Banana and cashews
- Chocolate-covered almonds and melon
- Granola and yogurt
- Hummus and pita chips
- Guacamole and tortilla chips

- Graham crackers with peanut butter
- Chocolate chip cookie and milk
- Banana bread and milk
- Ice cream bar and strawberries

Three-Item Snacks
- Apple, peanut butter, and milk
- Nuts (two servings) and dried fruit
- Energy bar, grapes, and juice
- Banana, cashews, and yogurt
- Chocolate-covered almonds (two servings) and banana
- Granola, yogurt, and berries
- Hummus, pita chips, and juice
- Guacamole, tortilla chips, and juice
- Graham crackers and peanut butter (two servings)
- Two chocolate chip cookies and milk
- Banana bread, milk, and nuts
- Ice cream bar, strawberries, and milk

Four-Item Snacks
- Apple, peanut butter (two servings), and milk
- Trail mix (two servings) and dried fruit (two servings)
- Energy bar, melon, yogurt, and juice
- Banana, cashews (two servings), and yogurt
- Chocolate-covered almonds (two servings), banana, and milk
- Granola, yogurt, berries, and nuts
- Hummus, pita chips (two servings), and juice
- Guacamole (two servings), tortilla chips, and juice
- Graham crackers (two servings) and peanut butter (two servings)
- Homemade ice cream sandwich (two chocolate chip cookies and vanilla ice cream) and milk
- Banana bread, nuts, and sixteen ounces of milk
- Ice cream bar, nuts, and sixteen ounces of juice

Special Circumstances

Getting sick can be very disorienting for a child with an eating disorder. Whether it's due to a stomach virus or a fever, your child's appetite will likely be off, which might alter their success with meals. The goal in this situation is for your child to do the best they can in the face of their illness. It might mean that the plate doesn't have all food groups present, or that you provide more fluids such as soups, juice, popsicles, and smoothies, and that's okay. Experiment with foods and fluids your child *can* eat while sick, encourage intake of as much volume as is tolerable, and once better, get back on track as soon as possible. The first few days after an illness might be difficult for your child as their metabolism becomes acclimated to adequate meals and snacks. The expectation is that, while uncomfortable, your child *can* complete meals and snacks and prolonging this step is likely to compromise recovery. It is also important that you notify the treatment team that your child is ill. The medical provider may want them to come in for a weight and vital-signs check to ensure they are not becoming medically unstable due to illness.

There may also be religious events that involve altering the diet. Those who are Catholic may avoid meat on Ash Wednesday and on Fridays during Lent. Muslims who follow Ramadan will fast from dawn to sunset for a month, and fasting is common for those who are Jewish on Yom Kippur and on other fast days throughout the year. When going through eating-disorder treatment, we suggest that your child be excused from these events due to medical reasons. Once more stable, you and the treatment team can evaluate whether your child is ready to participate again. Participating will depend on whether:

- They are medically stable.
- Their recovery is solid. (Would an alteration in their diet derail them?)
- They are able to supplement meals before and after fasting to make up for the void.

Go with Your Gut

Like anything, practice makes perfect! With time, plating balanced, wholesome meals will get easier. You may wish to outline a meal schedule that can help you stay organized with grocery shopping while ensuring a rotation of foods are being served. At first, you might feel more confident by keeping the guidelines, food group charts, and final review questions handy. Though you are also encouraged to go with your gut: does the plate look like it's enough to accomplish the task of nourishing your child? If it does, it's likely sufficient. If it doesn't, add more food. The goal of course is to help your child recover, both mentally and physically.

CHAPTER 10

What to Do If Your Child Still Isn't Gaining Enough Weight

Accelerated Nutritional Rehabilitation

"My son is eating so much food and he isn't gaining weight, how is this possible?"

"I couldn't possibly feed my daughter what you are recommending because she is always so uncomfortable after meals!"

"I don't know what else to add to my child's plate to help them gain weight, it's completely full!"

WEIGHT GAIN IS necessary for many adolescents with eating disorders in order to achieve complete medical and psychological recovery. To accomplish this, your child will require a high amount of calories, more than any parent might guess intuitively. Adolescents whose weight is within their expected weight range may be able to skip this step of accelerated nutritional rehabilitation; however, the information in this chapter may still be useful. Athletes who are still engaging in physical activity while going through this process will likely need to start right here—where the caloric density of the plate is higher.

At this point you are familiar with the plate, its contents, and the daily struggles of feeding your child five or six times per day. By now, your child is eating more than you have seen in months—and yet, it could be they are still having trouble gaining more weight. You may be asking yourself, "How is this possible? What is going on here?"

Welcome to accelerated nutritional rehabilitation. This is the next step for parents who are feeding their child the standard plate (as described in chapters 8 and 9) but whose weight gain progress has stalled or whose requirements may have changed (e.g, due to added exercise). You are doing a fantastic job already of feeding your child, and this section will help provide ideas to increase your child's intake further.

Hidden Calorie Loss

You may be wondering whether you really need to keep adding to your child's meals. And you may wonder if your child's inability to gain weight means they don't *need* to gain weight. That is not likely. The minute your child began eating more, their body started to wake up. It said, "Hey! I have food coming in. This is great! I've got work to do!" And as hard as you have fought the eating disorder during this process, the body has been fighting harder. It wants every last calorie that your child consumes in order to turn on those dormant body systems again so it can begin to repair and rebuild itself. This requires an incredible amount of fuel. And by now, your child has started eating more than you may have ever seen them eat, even before they became sick. Your medically fragile twelve-year-old daughter may be eating more than your seventeen-year-old basketball-playing son. This is normal, and should be expected. The caloric cost of rebuilding, plus the cost of catch-up growth is high.

You might be wondering where all those calories could possibly be going. Is your child is secretly exercising, purging, or feeding their meals to the dog? Your team may be asking you these questions as well. These are reasonable questions, and we suggest that parents find out the answers. You will never know for sure, but you should be confident there is not a secret loss of calories or increase in energy expenditure working against you.

Case Example: Gabriela

Gabriela's family was frustrated that she wasn't gaining weight after several weeks of FBT. A review with the dietitian of Gabriela's energy intake versus energy expenditure had everyone scratching their heads, because it seemed like she should be gaining weight based on what she was eating. She denied secretive exercise, purging, or throwing away her food. However, due to her school schedule, she was eating a significant amount of her meals unsupervised. Morning snack, lunch, and afternoon snack were all happening at school, on her own. Gabriela's parents and treatment team trusted *her* but did not trust her eating disorder, and decided something needed to change.

The family considered pulling Gabriela from the soccer team in order to reduce her caloric needs. They were hesitant, though, because they didn't want her to have to explain why she had to stop to all of her teammates. Instead, the family decided that they would reimplement mealtime supervision. They had her eat with the school nurse for morning snack and lunch, and then her mother met her for afternoon snack. Gabriela was frustrated with this sudden increase in supervision, but it worked. She started to gain weight, despite no increase in the meal plan. Sometimes, when things don't make sense, something might be going on that warrants further exploration. Typically, in these perplexing situations, it makes the most sense to start by going back to the time it last worked.

Why Weight Gain May Be Naturally Difficult

Often, as refeeding continues, the body can become hypermetabolic: there is an increase in the metabolic rate, which increases your child's energy expenditure and calorie requirements, making weight gain more difficult. During refeeding, there is an increase in the food's thermogenic effect, which refers to the amount of calories a body needs to digest food. In a healthy individual, the body will burn an extra 10 percent of calories to digest food. But in those with anorexia, this number can exceed 30 percent by week four of treatment.[1] This physiological response to refeeding makes it challenging for your child to gain weight. And getting your child who is struggling with an eating disorder to gain weight is hard enough without the added barrier of an increasing metabolic rate.

Weight gain at the rate of one to two pounds per week is expected in the outpatient setting, with two to three pounds per week expected if the adolescent is in a higher level of care, such as a partial hospitalization program or an intensive outpatient program.[2] Studies have shown that the faster this process is accomplished, the better the prognosis.[3] If your child is not gaining, it can feel daunting at times and you may feel at a loss of how to proceed. Please don't fret, however; there are plenty of ways to promote this rate of weight gain effectively and efficiently, and we hope your questions will be answered in this chapter.

Adjusting Your Child's Plates

The first thing to do is take a look at your child's current food intake.

- Is your child eating three meals and two snacks per day? If so, it's likely time for a third snack.
- Are your child's plates full? Is there any blank space on the plate? Where there's space, there isn't food: add some color to that blank canvas.
- How about the types of food? Does what you're feeding your child feel "safe," for instance, plain chicken breast, plain pasta, steamed veggies? If so, where can you add in some sauces and fats? Perhaps a couple of chicken thighs instead of a chicken breast? Your child used

to love your chicken Parmesan? Go for it! How about veggies? We can all agree that buttered carrots are much yummier than plain ones.

If you are already doing these suggestions, great work! However, if your child is not gaining weight, then it's time to adjust their meals.

You might be nervous that an adjustment to your child's meal plan will freak your child out. Of course, that can happen, but this is a good time to remind your child that their body needs this, as evidenced by their vital signs, menstrual cycle, or hormone levels. Although it may feel scary at first, it will get easier with practice and time.

Following is a list of ideas to increase the caloric density of your child's plate. You do not need to make these changes all at once! You might start with one option and see if that helps build some traction toward weight gain, and add more strategies as needed. As your child's metabolism speeds up, more increases will likely be necessary. As your child eats more, their body also burns more calories, making it difficult to gain weight.

- **Add juices or an extra glass of milk.** Liquid is easily digestible and leaves the stomach quickly, reducing feelings of fullness. Drinks are usually well tolerated, making adding them a great strategy to try first. Your child may resist juices because they've read about "added sugar," but it can be much easier for your child to drink a glass of juice than to add more volume to the plate. You can add juices to all meals, then all meals and snacks, adding about 500 to 700 calories from that change alone, depending on how many extra cups you add. If your child is already doing this, top that glass off or pull out those larger glasses from the back of the cabinet.
- **Add more items to your child's snacks.** Frequent snacking can help offset the amount of food your child consumes in one sitting, making it easier for your child to be successful. By now you are probably having your child eat two or three snacks a day. If they are currently having two snacks, add a third. How big is each snack? If your child

is having two items at each snack, now is the time to boost that up to three items. If your child is already having three items, add a fourth!

- **Aim for a "heaping half."** Now it is time to create a *heaping* half plate of grains/starches. This heaping half plate should be a mound and not a flat surface. This enables you to increase the volume of grains/starches without altering the proportions of each food group.
- **Add an extra item to each meal.** You have been plating meals that contain all food groups: dairy, grains/starches, fruit, vegetables, fats. As you move through this phase, you can add an extra serving of a food group—any group—of your choosing. If the meal is chicken marsala (protein), angel hair pasta (grains), sautéed asparagus (with olive oil, vegetables/fats), and a glass of milk (dairy), you can add a buttered dinner roll (grains/fats).
- **Add dessert to all meals.** You can also decide to plate a full meal and add a dessert on the side.
- **Use flavored milk such as chocolate, vanilla, or strawberry instead of plain.** Or add Carnation instant-breakfast powder to milk with meals.
- **Choose more calorically dense meals.**
  - Try loaded quesadillas with chicken, sour cream, and guacamole.
  - Stuffed crepes or omelets can be a great way to get multiple food groups into an entrée. Add cheese, sautéed veggies, sausage, guacamole, sour cream, etc.
  - Lasagna is a great way to mix food groups into a more compact entrée.
- **Add more fats.**
  - Add cream-based sauces to pasta, potatoes, cooked veggies.
  - Serve mashed potatoes (made with cream and butter) instead of roasted potatoes.
  - Serve a twice-baked potato or a loaded potato (with sour cream, butter, and cheese).
  - Add oil or butter to rice or serve fried rice.
  - Use olive oil when cooking, and add more right before serving.
  - Add avocado, mayo, and cheese to deli sandwiches.

- Double up on peanut butter in a PB&J sandwich.
- Add melted cheese to veggies.
- Use whole milk products instead of reduced-fat.
- **Add more calorically dense snacks.**
  - Serve ice cream for an evening snack.
  - Dense oatmeal bars or cookies can make a great snack.
- **Add a meal supplement.** Adding a supplement such as Ensure Plus, BOOST Plus, or any generic version of these, can be an easy and quick way to add calories. Because these shakes are nutrient dense, they will not take up a lot of space in your child's stomach. You can add one shake, two, or however many you think will be beneficial to your child. What's nice about an added shake is that they are very easy to remove once your child is ready for the next phase, weight maintenance.
- **Add smoothies or milk shakes.** This is where you, as a parent get to become creative in the kitchen. Smoothies are a great way to combine food groups into liquid form, which reduces volume. Listed below are a few recipes to get you started, however, it is just as easy to add whatever you have around at home into the blender. Ingredients that taste good together are generally dairy, fruit, and juices. You can also add ice cream or sherbet to increase the caloric density.

Milk Shake and Smoothie Recipes

Many smoothie and milkshake recipes are readily available online. Typically, these recipes include a dairy (milk, yogurt, or ice cream) blended with fruit of your choice (berries, bananas, peaches, and mango all work great). You can even try frozen fruit, which is cheaper and easier to keep on hand. Here are some ideas to get you started.

- **Mixed fruit smoothie:** Blend a handful each of strawberries, blueberries, pineapple, and mango; 1/2 cup whole milk yogurt; 1 cup whole milk, and ice.

- **Banana-chocolate smoothie:** Blend 1/2 banana, 2 tablespoons peanut butter, a few squirts of chocolate syrup, 1 cup whole milk, and ice.
- **Strawberry milk shake:** Blend 1/2 cup premium vanilla ice cream, a handful of strawberries, 1 cup whole milk, and ice.

For more information on how these additions translate into a day's eating, please see the following table, which provides examples of how to adjust the "standard" plate to be more calorically dense. Please note, while it is not advised to measure out foods at home, measurements are listed below for reference. These should be considered approximations and it is okay to give your child a little more or a little less as long as the food groups are met and the plate looks full.

Table 1. Plate-by-Plate Adjustments

MEAL	STANDARD	ADDED DRINKS	ACCELERATED
BREAKFAST	2 eggs, scrambled 2 slices toast with 1 tablespoon butter 1 cup fruit or 1 medium whole fruit 8 oz. 2 percent or whole milk	2 eggs, scrambled 2 slices toast with 1 tablespoon butter 1 cup fruit or 1 medium whole fruit 16 oz. 2 percent or whole milk	2 eggs, scrambled with ¼ cup shredded cheese 2 slices toast with 2 tablespoons butter fruit smoothie or milk shake 8 oz. whole milk
SNACK	6–8 oz. 2 percent or whole yogurt ¼ cup granola (morning snack is optional, depending on meal plan)	6–8 oz. 2 percent or whole yogurt ¼ cup granola 8 oz. apple juice	6–8 oz. 2 percent or whole yogurt ½ cup granola ¼ cup slivered almonds or coconut flakes 16 oz. apple juice

MEAL	STANDARD	ADDED DRINKS	ACCELERATED
LUNCH	Turkey sandwich: 2 slices bread 3 slices turkey 1 slice cheese 1 tablespoon mayo lettuce, tomato 1 serving pretzels 1 cup grapes	Turkey sandwich: 2 slices bread 3 slices turkey 1 slice cheese 1 tablespoon mayo lettuce, tomato 1 serving pretzels 1 cup grapes 8 oz. lemonade	Turkey sandwich: 2 slices bread 3 slices turkey 2 slices cheese 1 tablespoon mayo lettuce, tomato 1 ½ servings potato chips 1 cup grapes 16 oz. lemonade
SNACK	1 serving of pita chips ¼ cup hummus	1 serving of pita chips ¼ cup hummus 8 oz. 2 percent or whole milk	1 ½ servings of pita chips ¼ cup hummus smoothie or milk shake
DINNER	4–5 oz. barbecue chicken 1 cup rice pilaf 1 cup green beans with 1 tablespoon butter 8 oz. 2 percent or whole milk	4–5 oz. barbecue chicken 1 cup rice pilaf 1 cup green beans with 1 tablespoon butter 16 oz. 2 percent milk	4–5 oz. barbecue chicken 1 cup rice pilaf 1 cup green beans with 1 tablespoon butter 1 dinner roll with 1 tablespoon butter 16 oz. whole milk
SNACK	½ cup regular ice cream 1 cup raspberries	½ cup regular ice cream 1 cup raspberries 8 oz. cranberry juice	½ cup premium ice cream 1 cup raspberries 2 tablespoon chocolate chips 16 oz. whole milk
TOTAL CALORIES	**Approximately 2,600 (3 meals and 2 snacks)** **Approximately 2,800 (3 meals and 3 snacks)**	**Approximately 3,600**	**Approximately 4,500 (no shakes)** **Approximately 4,750 (one shake)** **Approximately 5,000 (two shakes)**

While the accelerated plate will be enough for many teens to gain weight, there is still the possibility that it will not be enough for your child. In this case, as long as no other weight gain-interfering behaviors are at play, you will need to continue to incrementally increase your child's plate until you find the right balance to promote weight gain. Your child *can* and *will* gain weight; however, it can take many rounds of adjustments to achieve and your team, specifically your dietician, can help guide you.

If, at this point, you are running out of ideas to increase your child's food intake and you feel you've reached the limit of their ability to consume the amount of food they need to gain weight, it's a good time to take a look at their activity level. If your child is doing a lot of physical activity, it may be necessary to reduce or eliminate activity until your child is able to gain weight. This will reduce the energy your child is expending in order to allow them to gain weight more easily.

Finally, if your child is not exercising and still unable to gain weight, as discussed before, it might be time to explore whether there are other behaviors at play. Are they purging, hiding food, using laxatives? It is important to remain curious whenever something doesn't seem to add up. Discuss this with your treatment team and allow them to help you investigate the current state of your child's eating disorder recovery.

Dealing with Stomach Pain Associated with Refeeding

While your child may be getting enough food at this point, it is likely that they are complaining about the amount they have to eat and/or how uncomfortable they feel. If your child is complaining of constipation, gas, and bloating, they are not alone. It is common for individuals struggling with eating disorders to complain of a wide variety of gastrointestinal-related issues. You may even be wondering if they are gluten-intolerant or lactose-intolerant. There can be some initial sensitivity to lactose, or foods that are high in fat, since malnutrition causes a suppression of the enzymes used to break these foods down. This will resolve and gets better with time. If your child was not lactose- or gluten-intolerant before the onset of their eating disorder, it is highly unlikely they are now. The best thing you can do for your child is to feed them a wide variety and balance of foods and food groups without avoiding anything they used to tolerate. These symptoms of gastrointestinal distress will resolve with time, consistency, and nourishment. It will take time for their body to rebuild and repair this very delicate system and in the meantime, you can expect to hear about it.

Some individuals do find temporary relief of symptoms through use of over-the-counter supplements such as probiotics, lactase enzymes, and antacids. Use of such supplements should be used conservatively and discussed with your child's treatment team. While they are generally considered harmless, the message it can send to your child and their eating disorder is that they *need* these supplements in order to eat normally, which will not be true as their bodies become nourished.

It may also be the case that what your child is eating is contributing to their digestive issues. Take a look at the following list of gas-producing foods. If your child is eating these regularly, it may be worth a trial of elimination or reduction of these foods from their diet.

- Beans (presoaking reduces the gas-producing potential of beans if you discard the soaking water and cook using fresh water)
- Vegetables such as artichokes, asparagus, broccoli, cabbage, brussels sprouts, cauliflower, cucumbers, green peppers, onions, radishes, celery, carrots
- Fruits such as apples, peaches, raisins, bananas, apricots, prune juice, pears
- Whole grains and bran (adding them slowly to your diet can help reduce gas-forming potential)
- Carbonated drinks (allowing carbonated drinks, which contain a great deal of gas, to stand open for several hours allows the carbonation/gas to escape)
- Foods containing sorbitol, such as dietetic foods and sugar-free candies and gums[4]

In general, the more roughage in the diet, the more symptoms of gas and bloating your child will experience. Remember, their digestive tract is weak right now and it will take time for it to rebuild its strength. Easy-to-digest foods with fewer fruits and vegetables will allow your child to consume adequate nutrition without the extra discomfort.

Weight Gain: A New Body and New Clothes

During this phase of nutritional rehabilitation, when weight gain is the priority, your child will likely become distressed by the changes they see and perceive happening with their body. As will be discussed in chapter 12, talking about weight with your child is not advised. However, your child will notice their body changing and will need your support and encouragement. It is normal for your child to gain weight primarily around their face and abdomen initially, which can be very upsetting, though the weight eventually disperses more evenly throughout the body.

Engaging in weight conversations doesn't help and will only go in circles. Your child will need your loving support. Remind them that these changes are necessary and that their body is doing what it needs to. Encourage your child to trust this process and to be patient while their body achieves balance and stability. Your child will also need new clothes at this point, a task you have likely been dreading. Shopping can either be a source of great pleasure or a fraught experience for anyone depending on their relationship with their body. And for a teenager recovering from an eating disorder, it will likely be the latter.

Parents may sometimes feel worried about their child's new body. Some may wonder if their child has gained too much weight. Normalizing how one eats and going from a place of dieting to a place of nourishment might require some weight gain to occur during recovery. Linda Bacon, PhD, researcher and author of *Body Respect* and *Health at Every Size*, says that if parents are concerned that their child is now "fat" they might be tempted to support an attitude of restraint. Kids who are recovering from an eating disorder need support from their parents and help boosting their self-esteem. Dr. Bacon advises, "Reinforce the idea that kids come in a wide range of sizes and that every body is a good body . . . fat or thin, when kids are taught to appreciate, not hate, themselves, it will support them in making better choices." Your child's weight will need time to settle, so Dr. Bacon encourages you to help your child focus on behavior and attitude rather than on weight.

How do I buy my child new clothes without them having a complete meltdown? What if handing them new clothes causes them to refuse to eat? These are great questions, and there are several ways to thread this needle that can help avoid a disaster. We have outlined ten key steps to ensure that you and your child complete this necessary task successfully.

1. Talk to your child about shopping when they are calm and well rested.
2. Consider having this discussion during a family-based treatment session so that the therapist can help facilitate a healthy conversation and provide skills for your child to use if they become distressed.
3. Let your child know, in a firm and loving way, that you are planning to shop for new clothes for them and ask if they want to be a part of this process.
4. If your child does want to be involved, ask them how they imagine it will go. Will it be fun? Or are they nervous, and worried about becoming overwhelmed? If they imagine the latter, offer to do the shopping for them and talk about what types of clothes they might want.
5. Take stock of what your child currently has in their closet and drawers. What fits and has room for growth? What doesn't fit?
6. Anything that doesn't fit should be donated. Your child may beg to hang on to some of their clothes that fit them when they were at

their lowest weight. Let them know that you are not going to keep "sick" clothes because it won't allow them to continue to move forward in their recovery.

7. Do not hand down the clothes your child fit into when they were malnourished to their younger siblings, cousins, or friends. This will lead your child to feel jealous that others get to be that weight, yet they can't. It will be difficult for your child to see other people in their community wearing their old clothes, which serves as another reminder that they are now living in a larger body. Instead, consider donating them or throwing them away. Your child should never have to see those clothes again.

8. During the recovery process, your child may be highly sensitive to the feeling of the waistband in their clothing. Consider buying stretchy, breathable, and loose pants instead of the ever-popular "skinny" jeans. Breezy dresses without a waistline will feel better to your child than formfitting dresses. There are many fashionable options for clothes that can help your child feel more comfortable during this phase.

9. Remember, your child will eventually be able to wear tighter clothing and feel comfortable in them, though this will take time.

10. If your child is joining you on the shopping trip, consider buying a few new weight-neutral options—fun socks, a new necklace, or a hat. These are options your child can get excited about while taking the focus off size.

MEAL PLAN
Standard Plates: Three Meals and Two to Three Snacks

MEAL		1	2	3	
Breakfast	Starch	Oatmeal	Toast (2 slices)	Pancakes	
	Protein	Nuts	Eggs	Breakfast sausage	
	Vegetable/Fruit	Apple	Banana	Orange	
	Fat	Butter	Butter	Butter	
	Dairy	Milk	Yogurt	Yogurt	
	Other/Side	Brown sugar		Syrup	
Snack	Two items	Yogurt Granola	Crackers Cheese	Muffin Nuts	
Lunch	Starch	Turkey sandwich	Pizza (2 slices)	Ham sandwich	
	Protein	(Turkey in sandwich)	(Cheese on pizza)	(Ham on sandwich)	
	Vegetable/Fruit	Lettuce/tomato, pear	Mixed salad	Grapes	
	Fat	Avocado	Salad dressing	Mayonnaise	
	Dairy	Cheese	Milk	Cheese	
	Other/Side	Pretzels		Chips	
Snack	Two items	Hummus Pita chips	Guacamole Tortilla chips	Crackers Cheese	
Dinner	Starch	Rice	Pesto pasta	Tortillas	
	Protein	Chicken	Salmon	Steak fajitas	
	Vegetable/Fruit	Asparagus	Broccoli	Bell peppers/onion	
	Fat	Oil	(Pesto on pasta)	Sour cream	
	Dairy	Milk	Parmesan cheese	Shredded cheese	
Snack	Two items	Cookies Milk	Fruit smoothie Graham crackers	Ice cream Mixed berries	

The Plate-by-Plate Approach

4	5	6	7
Granola	English muffin	Bagel	Cereal, toast
Yogurt	Eggs	Eggs	Bacon
Blueberries	Banana	Strawberries	Pear
Nuts	Avocado	Cream cheese	Butter
Milk	Cheese	Milk	Milk
Trail mix Juice	Granola bar Milk	Brownie Milk	Chips Guacamole
Grilled cheese	PB&J sandwich	Wrap	Hot dog bun
(Cheese in sandwich)	(Peanut butter)	Chicken	Hot dog
Tomato soup	Apple	Lettuce, cucumber	Grapes
Butter	Cookie	Hummus	Potato chips
Milk	Milk	Feta cheese	Milk
	(Jelly)	Pita chips	
Cookie Milk	Yogurt Granola	Nature Valley bar Juice	Chocolate-covered dried fruit Yogurt
Couscous	Spaghetti, garlic bread	Lo mein	Hamburger bun
BBQ Chicken	Meatballs	Chicken teriyaki	Burger
Sautéed spinach	Green beans	Stir-fried mixed veggies	Salad
Oil	Butter	Oil	Salad dressing, avocado
Milk	Parmesan cheese	Milk	Cheese
Chocolate Nuts	Toast Peanut butter	Chocolate-covered almonds Dried mango	Yogurt Granola

MEAL PLAN
Vegetarian Plates: Three Meals and Two to Three Snacks

MEAL		1	2	3	
Breakfast	Starch	Oatmeal	Toast (2 slices)	Pancakes	
	Protein	Nuts	Eggs	Veggie sausage	
	Vegetable/Fruit	Apple	Banana	Orange	
	Fat	Butter	Butter	Butter	
	Dairy	Milk	Yogurt	Yogurt	
	Other/Side	Brown sugar		Syrup	
Snack	Two items	Yogurt Granola	Crackers Cheese	Muffin Nuts	
Lunch	Starch	Cheese sandwich	Pizza (2 slices)	Hamburger bun	
	Protein	Hummus	(Cheese on pizza)	Veggie burger	
	Vegetable/Fruit	Lettuce/tomato, pear	Mixed salad	Lettuce/tomato	
	Fat	Avocado	Salad dressing	Mayonnaise, avocado	
	Dairy	Cheese	Milk	Cheese	
	Other/Side	Pretzels		Chips	
Snack	Two items	Hummus Pita chips	Guacamole Tortilla chips	Crackers Cheese	
Dinner	Starch	Stir-fried rice	Pesto pasta	Tortillas	
	Protein	Tofu, egg (in rice)	Milk	Beans	
	Vegetable/Fruit	Stir-fried mixed veggies	Broccoli	Bell peppers/onion	
	Fat	Oil	(Pesto on pasta)	Sour cream	
	Dairy	Milk	Parmesan cheese	Shredded cheese	
Snack	Two items	Cookies Milk	Fruit smoothie Graham crackers	Ice cream Mixed berries	

The Plate-by-Plate Approach

4	5	6	7
Granola	English muffin	Bagel	Cereal, toast
Yogurt	Eggs	Eggs	Veggie bacon
Blueberries	Banana	Strawberries	Pear
Nuts	Avocado	Cream cheese	Butter
Milk	Cheese	Milk	Milk
Trail mix Juice	Granola bar Milk	Brownie Milk	Chips Guacamole
Grilled cheese	PB&J sandwich	Wrap	Hot dog bun
(Cheese in sandwich)	(Peanut butter)	Falafel	Veggie sausage
Tomato soup	Apple	Lettuce, cucumber	Grapes
Butter	Cookie	Hummus	Potato chips
MIlk	Milk	Feta cheese	Milk
	(Jelly)	Pita chips	
Cookie Milk	Yogurt Granola	Nature Valley bar Juice	Chocolate-covered dried fruit Yogurt
Couscous	Spaghetti, garlic bread	Lo mein	Hamburger bun
Fried tofu	Veggie meatballs	Tofu teriyaki, edamame beans	Veggie burger
Sautéed spinach	Green beans	Stir-fried mixed veggies	Salad
Oil	Butter	Oil	Salad dressing, avocado
Milk	Parmesan cheese	Milk	Cheese
Chocolate Nuts	Toast Peanut butter	Chocolate-covered almonds Dried mango	Yogurt Granola

MEAL PLAN
Standard Plates: Three Meals and Two to Three Snacks + Drinks

MEAL		1	2	3	
Breakfast	Starch	Oatmeal	Toast (2 slices)	Pancakes	
	Protein	Nuts	Eggs	Breakfast sausage	
	Vegetable/Fruit	Apple	Banana	Orange	
	Fat	Butter	Butter	Butter	
	Dairy	Milk	Yogurt	Yogurt	
	Other/Side	Brown sugar		Syrup	
	Drink	Additional cup of milk	Juice	Juice	
Snack	Two items Drink	Yogurt Granola Juice	Crackers Cheese Juice	Muffin Nuts Milk	
Lunch	Starch	Turkey sandwich	Pizza (2 slices)	Ham sandwich	
	Protein	(Turkey in sandwich)	(Cheese on pizza)	(Ham on sandwich)	
	Vegetable/Fruit	Lettuce/tomato, pear	Mixed salad	Grapes	
	Fat	Avocado	Salad dressing	Mayonnaise	
	Dairy	Cheese	Milk	Cheese	
	Other/Side	Pretzels		Chips	
	Drink	Juice	Additional cup of milk	Juice	
Snack	Two items Drink	Hummus Pita chips Juice	Guacamole Tortilla chips Juice	Crackers Cheese Juice	
Dinner	Starch	Rice	Pesto pasta	Tortillas	
	Protein	Chicken	Salmon	Steak fajitas	
	Vegetable/Fruit	Asparagus	Broccoli	Bell peppers/onion	
	Fat	Oil	(Pesto on pasta)	Sour cream	
	Dairy	Milk	Parmesan cheese	Shredded cheese	
	Other/Side				
	Drink	Additional cup of milk	Juice	Juice	
Snack	Two items Drink	Cookies Milk (2 servings, for added drink)	Graham crackers Fruit smoothie (2 servings, for added drink)	Ice cream Mixed berries Juice	

The Plate-by-Plate Approach

4	5	6	7
Granola	English muffin	Bagel	Cereal and toast
Yogurt	Eggs	Eggs	Bacon
Blueberries	Banana	Strawberries	Pear
Nuts	Avocado	Cream cheese	Butter
Milk	Cheese	Milk	Milk
Additional cup of milk	Juice	Additional cup of milk	Additional cup of milk
Trail mix Juice (2 servings, for added drink)	Granola bar Milk (2 servings, for added drink)	Brownie Milk (2 servings, for added drink)	Chips Guacamole Juice
Grilled cheese	PB&J sandwich	Wrap	Hot dog bun
(Cheese in sandwich)	(Peanut butter)	Chicken	Hot dog
Tomato soup	Apple	Lettuce, cucumber	Grapes
Butter	Cookie	Hummus	Potato chips
Milk	Milk	Feta cheese	Milk
	(Jelly)	Pita chips	
Additional cup of milk	Additional cup of milk	Juice	Additional cup of milk
Cookie Milk (2 servings, for added drink)	Yogurt Granola Juice	Nature Valley bar Juice (2 servings, for added drink)	Chocolate-covered dried fruit Yogurt Juice
Couscous	Spaghetti, garlic bread	Lo mein	Hamburger bun
BBQ Chicken	Meatballs	Chicken teriyaki	Burger
Sautéed spinach	Green beans	Stir-fried mixed veggies	Salad
Oil	Butter	Oil	Salad dressing, avocado
Milk	Parmesan cheese	Milk	Cheese
Additional cup of milk	Juice	Additional cup of milk	Juice
Chocolate Nuts Milk	Toast Peanut butter Milk	Chocolate-covered almonds Dried mango Juice	Yogurt Granola Juice

MEAL PLAN
Vegetarian Plates: Three Meals and Two to Three Snacks + Drinks

MEAL		1	2	3	
Breakfast	Starch	Oatmeal	Toast (2 slices)	Pancakes	
	Protein	Nuts	Eggs	Veggie sausage	
	Vegetable/Fruit	Apple	Banana	Orange	
	Fat	Butter	Butter	Butter	
	Dairy	Milk	Yogurt	Yogurt	
	Other/Side	Brown sugar		Syrup	
	Drink	Additional cup of milk	Juice	Juice	
Snack	Two items / Drink	Yogurt / Granola / Juice	Crackers / Cheese / Juice	Muffin / Nuts / Milk	
Lunch	Starch	Cheese sandwich	Pizza (2 slices)	Hamburger bun	
	Protein	Hummus	(Cheese on pizza)	Veggie burger	
	Vegetable/Fruit	Lettuce/tomato, pear	Mixed salad	Lettuce/tomato	
	Fat	Avocado	Salad dressing	Mayonnaise, avocado	
	Dairy	Cheese	Milk	Cheese	
	Other/Side	Pretzels		Chips	
	Drink	Juice	Additional cup of milk	Juice	
Snack	Two items / Drink	Hummus / Pita chips / Juice	Guacamole / Tortilla chips / Juice	Crackers / Cheese / Juice	
Dinner	Starch	Stir-fried rice	Pesto pasta	Tortillas	
	Protein	Tofu, egg (in rice)	Milk	Beans	
	Vegetable/Fruit	Stir-fried mixed veggies	Broccoli	Bell peppers/onion	
	Fat	Oil	(Pesto on pasta)	Sour cream	
	Dairy	Milk	Parmesan cheese	Shredded cheese	
	Drink	Additional cup of milk	Additional cup of milk	Juice	
Snack	Two items / Drink	Cookies / Milk (2 servings, for added drink)	Graham crackers / Fruit smoothie (2 servings, for added drink)	Ice cream / Mixed berries / Juice	

The Plate-by-Plate Approach

4	5	6	7
Granola	English muffin	Bagel	Cereal, toast
Yogurt	Eggs	Eggs	Veggie bacon
Blueberries	Banana	Strawberries	Pear
Nuts	Avocado	Cream cheese	Butter
Milk	Cheese	Milk	Milk
Additional cup of milk	Juice	Additional cup of milk	Additional cup of milk
Trail mix Juice (2 servings, for added drink)	Granola bar Milk (2 servings, for added drink)	Brownie Milk (2 servings, for added drink)	Chips Guacamole Juice
Grilled cheese	PB&J sandwich	Wrap	Hot dog bun
(Cheese in sandwich)	(Peanut butter)	Falafel	Veggie sausage
Tomato soup	Apple	Lettuce, cucumber	Grapes
Butter	Cookie	Hummus	Potato chips
Milk	Milk	Feta cheese	Milk
	(Jelly)	Pita chips	
Additional cup of milk	Additional cup of milk	Juice	Additional cup of milk
Cookie Milk (2 servings, for added drink)	Yogurt Granola Juice	Nature Valley bar Juice (2 servings, for added drink)	Chocolate-covered dried fruit Yogurt Juice
Couscous	Spaghetti, garlic bread	Lo mein	Hamburger bun
Fried tofu	Veggie meatballs	Tofu teriyaki, edamame beans	Veggie burger
Sautéed spinach	Green beans	Stir-fried mixed veggies	Salad
Oil	Butter	Oil	Salad dressing, avocado
Milk	Parmesan cheese	Milk	Cheese
Additional cup of milk	Juice	Additional cup of milk	Juice
Chocolate Nuts Milk	Toast Peanut butter Milk	Chocolate-covered almonds Dried mango Juice	Yogurt Granola Juice

MEAL PLAN
Accelerated Plates: Three Meals and Three Snacks (3 items each) + Drinks + 2 Shakes

MEAL		1	2	3	
Breakfast	Starch	Oatmeal, toast	Toast (3 slices)	Pancakes	
	Protein	Nuts	Eggs	Breakfast sausage	
	Vegetable/ Fruit	Apple	Banana	Orange	
	Fat	Butter, peanut butter	Butter	Butter	
	Dairy	Milk	Yogurt	Yogurt	
	Other/Side	Brown sugar	Jam	Syrup	
	Drink	Additional cup milk	Juice (2 cups)	Shake	
Snack	Three items Drink	Yogurt Granola Nuts Juice	Crackers Cheese Salami Juice	Muffin Nuts Banana Milk	
Lunch	Starch	Turkey sandwich	Pizza (3 slices)	Ham sandwich	
	Protein	(Turkey in sandwich)	(Cheese on pizza)	(Ham on sandwich)	
	Vegetable/ Fruit	Lettuce/tomato, pear	Mixed salad	Grapes	
	Fat	Avocado, mayo	Salad dressing	Mayonnaise, avocado	
	Dairy	Cheese (2 servings)	(Milk in shake)	Cheese (2 servings)	
	Other/Side	Pretzels		Chips	
	Drink	Shake	Shake	Shake	
Snack	Three items Drink	Hummus Pita chips Cheese Juice	Guacamole Tortilla chips Juice (2 servings, for added drink)	Crackers Cheese Salami Juice	
Dinner	Starch	Rice, bread roll	Pesto pasta, bread	Tortillas	
	Protein	Chicken	Salmon	Steak fajitas	
	Vegetable/ Fruit	Asparagus	Broccoli	Bell peppers/onion	
	Fat	Oil, butter	(Pesto on pasta), butter	Sour cream, guacamole	
	Dairy	(Milk in shake)	Parmesan cheese	Shredded cheese	
	Other/Side			Tortilla chips	
	Drink	Shake	Shake	Juice	
Snack	Three items Drink	Cookies Nuts Milk (2 servings, for added drink)	Graham crackers Peanut butter Fruit smoothie (2 servings, for added drink)	Premium ice cream Mixed berries Whipped cream Juice (2 servings, for added drink)	

The Plate-by-Plate Approach

4	5	6	7
Granola, toast	English muffins (2 servings)	Bagel	Cereal, toast (2 slices)
Yogurt	Eggs	Eggs	Bacon
Blueberries	Banana	Strawberries	Pear
Nuts	Avocado	Cream cheese	Butter
(Milk in shake)	Cheese (2 servings)	(Milk in shake)	(Milk in shake)
Butter, jam	Butter		Jam
Shake	Juice (2 cups)	Shake	Shake
Trail mix Yogurt Juice (2 servings, for added drink)	Granola bar Apple, peanut butter Milk (2 servings, for added drink)	2 brownies Milk (2 servings, for added drink)	Chips Guacamole Juice (2 servings, for added drink)
Grilled cheese	PB&J sandwich	Wrap	Hot dog bun
(Cheese in sandwich)	(Peanut butter)	Chicken	Hot dog
Tomato soup	Apple	Lettuce, cucumber	Grapes
Butter	Cookies	Hummus, avocado	Potato chips
Milk (in shake)	(Milk in shake)	Feta cheese, yogurt	(Milk in shake)
	(Jelly), sliced cheese	Pita chips	Baked beans
Shake	Shake	Juice	Shake
Cookies Nuts Milk (2 servings, for added drink)	Yogurt Granola Chocolate chips Juice	Nature Valley bar Banana Nuts Shake	Chocolate-covered dried fruit Yogurt Banana Juice
Couscous, bread	Spaghetti, garlic bread	Lo mein	Hamburger bun
BBQ Chicken	Meatballs	Chicken teriyaki	Burger
Sautéed spinach	Green beans	Stir-fried mixed veggies	Salad
Oil, butter	Butter	Oil	Salad dressing, avocado
(Milk in shake)	Parmesan cheese	Milk	Cheese
		Pot stickers	French fries
Shake	Juice	Additional cup of milk	Juice
Chocolate Nuts Dried apricots Milk	Toast Peanut butter Banana Shake	Chocolate-covered almonds Dried mango Animal crackers Milk	Yogurt Granola Nuts Juice

MEAL PLAN
Accelerated Vegetarian Plates: Three Meals and Three Snacks (3 items each) + Drinks + 2 Shakes

MEAL		1	2	3	
Breakfast	Starch	Oatmeal, toast	Toast (3 slices)	Pancakes	
	Protein	Nuts	Eggs	Veggie sausage	
	Vegetable/Fruit	Apple	Banana	Orange	
	Fat	Butter, peanut butter	Butter	Butter	
	Dairy	Milk	Yogurt	Yogurt	
	Other/Side	Brown sugar	Jam	Syrup	
	Drink	Additional cup of milk	Juice (2 servings)	Shake	
Snack	Three items / Drink	Yogurt Granola Nuts Juice	Crackers Cheese Avocado Juice	Muffin Nuts Banana Milk	
Lunch	Starch	Cheese sandwich	Pizza (3 slices)	Hamburger bun	
	Protein	Hummus	(Cheese on pizza)	Veggie burger	
	Vegetable/Fruit	Lettuce/tomato, pear	Mixed salad	Lettuce/tomato	
	Fat	Avocado	Salad dressing	Mayonnaise, avocado	
	Dairy	Cheese (2 servings)	(Milk in shake)	Cheese (2 servings)	
	Other/Side	Pretzels		Chips	
	Drink	Shake	Shake	Shake	
Snack	Three items / Drink	Hummus Pita chips Cheese Juice	Guacamole Tortilla chips Juice (2 servings, for added drink)	Crackers Cheese Avocado Juice	
Dinner	Starch	Stir-fried rice, egg rolls	Pesto pasta, bread	Tortillas	
	Protein	Tofu, egg (in rice)	(Milk in shake)	Beans	
	Vegetable/Fruit	Stir-fried mixed veggies	Broccoli	Bell peppers/onion	
	Fat	Oil	(Pesto in pasta), butter	Sour cream, guacamole	
	Dairy	Milk (in shake)	Parmesan cheese	Shredded cheese	
	Other/Side			Tortilla chips	
	Drink	Shake	Shake	Juice	
Snack	Three items / Drink	Cookies Nuts Milk (2 servings, for added drink)	Graham crackers Peanut butter Fruit smoothie (2 servings, for added drink)	Premium ice cream Mixed berries Whipped cream Juice (2 servings, for added drink)	

4	5	6	7
Granola, toast	English muffins (2 servings)	Bagel	Cereal, toast (2 slices)
Yogurt	Eggs	Eggs	Veggie bacon
Blueberries	Banana	Strawberries	Pear
Nuts	Avocado	Cream cheese	Butter
(Milk in shake)	Cheese (2 servings)	(Milk in shake)	(Milk in shake)
Butter, jam	Butter		Jam
Shake	Juice (2 servings)	Shake	Shake
Trail mix Yogurt Juice (2 servings, for added drink)	Granola bar Apple, peanut butter Milk (2 servings, for added drink)	2 brownies Milk (2 servings, for added drink	Chips Guacamole Juice (2 servings, for added drink)
Grilled cheese	PB&J sandwich	Wrap	Hot dog bun
(Cheese in sandwich)	(Peanut butter)	Falafel	Veggie sausage
Tomato soup	Apple	Lettuce, cucumber	Grapes
Butter	Cookies	Hummus, avocado	Potato chips
(Milk in shake)	(Milk in shake)	Feta cheese, yogurt	(Milk in shake)
	(Jelly), sliced cheese	Pita chips	Baked beans
Shake	Shake	Juice	Shake
Cookies Nuts Milk (2 servings, for added drink)	Yogurt Granola Chocolate chips Juice	Nature Valley bar Banana Nuts Shake	Chocolate-covered dried fruit Yogurt Banana Juice
Couscous	Spaghetti, garlic bread	Lo mein	Hamburger bun
Fried tofu	Veggie meatballs	Tofu teriyaki, edamame beans	Veggie burger
Sautéed spinach	Green beans	Stir-fried mixed veggies	Salad
Oil	Butter	Oil	Salad dressing, avocado
Milk	Parmesan cheese	Milk	Cheese
		Pot stickers	French fries
Additional cup of milk	Juice	Additional cup of milk	Juice
Chocolate Nuts Dried apricots Milk	Toast Peanut butter Banana Shake	Chocolate-covered almonds Dried mango Animal crackers Milk	Yogurt Granola Nuts Juice

PART III

Returning
to Normal

CHAPTER 11

Weight Maintenance, Adding Back Physical Activity, and Increasing Independence

Phase 2 of FBT

"When can this weight gain stop?"

"If my child keeps eating this much, won't they gain too much weight?"

"Soccer tryouts start next month, what do we do?"

CONTINUED WEIGHT GAIN will be necessary until your child nears or reaches their goal weight range. As they near this range, your treatment team will begin to adjust their intake and energy expenditure to establish weight stabilization or "maintenance." This will begin Phase 2 of family-based treatment. By this point, most of your child's weight gain has been accomplished, and the focus will shift to weight maintenance, adding back exercise if it hasn't been already, as well as some food autonomy.

Transition to Weight Maintenance

It is important to note that the term *maintenance* should be used carefully. With adults, maintenance is a true weight plateau. However, in children and adolescents, maintenance includes the expectation that they continue to grow and develop along their natural growth curve. Some individuals will begin their growth spurt at this stage, about to face rapid increases in both height and weight. For others, they might be nearing the end of their growth, transitioning to their young adult height and weight range.

This transition to weight maintenance is tricky. Your child may not want to hear that they are nearing their goal weight range; they may be very sensitive to this information as it means they have gained a significant amount of weight that they won't be allowed to lose again. They may interpret being in their goal weight range as synonymous with "being fat." They are adjusting to a body that feels uncomfortable and new, all while buying new and bigger clothes or giving up clothes that are too small for their weight-restored body. For these reasons, it is recommended that the topic of weight maintenance, exercise, and meal plan reductions be addressed carefully.

Since weight maintenance can be a sensitive subject for your child, we encourage families to refrain from commenting about weight and shape. Comments about weight and shape can be triggering for kids with eating disorders, and are easily misinterpreted. Comments from others such as "you look great" or "you look healthy" may translate to "They must *really* mean that I look fat." Some kids may hear those comments and think, "See, I look healthy, so I can stop gaining weight." For more information about this, refer to Chapter 12: How to Talk About Diet and Weight (Hint: Don't!).

Integrating Exercise

As your child reaches their goal weight range and their vital signs improve, the treatment team will begin to approve activity in small, structured doses. They will begin discussing with you and your child how to incorporate safe and appropriate exercise while maintaining treatment goals. Many important conversations should occur at this point. If your child was previously a competitive soccer player, do they want to return to soccer?

Maybe not—it can surprise parents to learn that their child's interests have shifted since treatment began. Perhaps their teammates weren't healthy themselves or there was a strong diet culture on the team. Or maybe, your child associates soccer with illness because they played soccer while in the depths of their eating disorder and going back feels too risky. If that's the case, your child may not want to return to soccer.

If a sport has lost its allure, and your child isn't interested in returning, don't force it. They will need to begin experimenting with what a full and happy life post–eating disorder looks like, and it may look very different than their pre-illness life. Your child may want to try out other sports or they may want to focus on a different kind of recreational activity. There are all kinds of fun activities that your child can add into their life—hiking, bowling, bike rides around town, casual tennis with a friend, salsa dancing, surfing, theater—these may be more appealing to your child now, who may appropriately be trying to protect the recovery they worked so hard to achieve.

Once you have identified which activities interest your child, physical activity will be added in slowly and gradually. In some ways it's akin to a child returning to sport after an injury. If your child tore their ACL, it would be a long, slow process to test the knee out to ensure it was ready for competition. If they experienced pain, they would likely need to adjust training parameters. If they felt good, and were able to continue adhering to treatment targets, it is likely that it would be appropriate to gradually increase their training. Similarly, the duration and intensity of exercise should start out light, and progress with time to something longer and harder, if appropriate and supported by your child's treatment team. Your child will need to learn to be mindful with their movement, so they can listen to their body cues, and stop when they're tired, or go slower than they are normally inclined to.

Your child's treatment team may first approve supervised walks, for fifteen minutes twice a week. As that is added back in successfully with continued medical stability, your child may be allowed to increase walks to thirty minutes three times a week. After demonstrating consistent adherence to less intense exercise, the team may support more intense exercise. If your child is a runner, they may be approved to jog (slowly and supervised) for ten or twenty minutes at a time. Or perhaps, they are a swimmer and are now approved to get back in the pool to swim laps for fifteen minutes (again slowly, and supervised).

The Importance of Rest

As discussed in Chapter 5: To Exercise or Not, rest is an important part of rebuilding a balanced relationship with exercise. Your child should plan to take frequent rest breaks during activity and will be advised to take rest days during the week as well. The team will want to check in with your child about whether they are able to stick to the agreed upon duration, intensity, and frequency of exercise and rest. If your child cannot stick to the plan, it may be a red flag that your child is not quite ready to incorporate fitness or to progress in their training at this time. It might also be a red flag if your child ignores cues from their body, for example, running through pain in their shins or difficulty breathing. If your child reverts back to training in an underfueled or dehydrated state, then exercise should be limited again until they are able to follow their treatment team's recommendations. And lastly, if there are any large changes in your child's medical status (weight or vital signs), exercise should be placed on hold.

Red Flags in Beginning a New Fitness Program

- Your child does not take rest days
- Your child exceeds the duration, intensity, or frequency of exercise agreed upon by the treatment team
- Your child is not in tune with their body, ignoring cues to stop or slow down
- Your child trains in an underfueled or dehydrated state
- Your child is losing weight
- Your child's vital signs become unstable

Exercise Avoidance

Once weight-restored, it is possible that your child who was pushing to exercise suddenly decides they are no longer interested in exercising at all. This "exercise avoidance" can happen because the child suddenly feels uncomfortable in their new body. They may be concerned about their thighs jiggling during movement, or dislike seeing how their stomach looks in their fitted tank top. Wearing tight exercise clothes, or a formfitting leotard or swimsuit, can be challenging for your child as they acclimate to physical changes.

Your child may avoid exercise because they are protective of their recovery. They may be concerned about jeopardizing what they have accomplished during treatment, so they decide they don't want to experiment with altering their meal plan or energy balance to begin activity. They may not feel particularly connected to any one type of activity; perhaps they don't want to "go to the gym" because it feels forced and isn't fun, but they don't know what else they want to do. This can be a good time to explore and experiment with different activities until your child finds the one that is most enjoyable. Some kids may feel scarred from a previously unbalanced relationship with exercise, they may feel burned out, and may just not feel like exercising at this time. Last, they may avoid exercise because they finally found balance, health, and appreciation for their body and they are concerned about again becoming compulsive with exercise. For now, they may wish to solidify their recovery for a little bit longer before shaking things up.

You might feel relieved that your child has decided to take a break from exercise. However, the complete avoidance of exercise can pose unique challenges and increase body image distress that could be a catalyst for previous eating-disorder behaviors to reemerge. As discussed in chapter 5, exercise can help with mood, long-term management of emotions, sleep, and provide positive socialization benefits. Both extremes, exercising excessively or avoiding it entirely, pose problems. Working with your child to develop a positive, balanced relationship with exercise that is fun, enjoyable, and occurs with realistic frequency is typically a good goal. However, it is not uncommon for this process to take time and require extensive support from parents and the treatment team.

Adjusting or Reducing Your Child's Food Intake

At this stage, you and your child are likely wondering how and when to adjust food intake due to the new goal of weight maintenance, and/or the addition of exercise.

If your child is now exercising, you may not need to reduce their plate volume. It takes an incredible amount of energy to fuel an athletic body, especially in the adolescent years, which are already notorious for increased energy demands. Rather than decrease your child's current meal plan to prepare for weight maintenance, adding exercise offsets that. The medical visits should still be occurring regularly and will provide valuable feedback on whether your child is in balance or not. If your child's weight stays stable, balance has most likely been achieved! However, if your child loses weight the first weeks in which exercise is added, you likely need to add more food to account for the increased activity.

If your child was not previously athletic or they are choosing not to return to a highly active lifestyle, their nutrition needs may decrease slightly as they reach their goal weight range. Remember all those tips for increasing your child's plate? The added drinks at all meals and snacks? The desserts, the larger mound of rice or pasta? Now is a good time to (cautiously) experiment with tapering down some of those additions. Please do not stop them all at once! Your child's body will still require a significant amount of nutrition to maintain their weight for normal growth and development. In fact, adolescence is naturally a time of high energy requirements. Even if your teen didn't ever develop an eating disorder, they would likely be eating more than you think they need, especially during a growth spurt. A typical teen would be asking for second helpings, and raiding the fridge or pantry after school. Try removing one thing at a time, ever so cautiously, in order to see how your child's body responds. Again, the medical visits will provide you with valuable feedback as to how the changes are working.

The following suggestions will help you carefully guide your child toward weight maintenance with a reduction in their meal plan. Some kids may only require one or two nutritional changes. Others may need several changes to achieve weight maintenance.

Tips for Decreasing Your Child's Plate

- **Make beverages optional.** Let your child know that due to their medical progress, their stability, and their efforts, the beverages they previously required at each meal and snack (e.g., juice or additional milk) can now be adjusted. You may wish to peel back the drinks at snacks first (taking away two or three cups of juice/additional milk to start), while leaving the drinks at meals. You can then make further adjustments as needed, and remove all drinks from meals (taking away another three cups of juice or additional milk). These drinks can now be "optional"; your child can choose to have it, or not, as long as their meals contain all the necessary food groups. If they do take away the added beverages, they will likely need to drink more water throughout the day to prevent dehydration.

- **Reduce the number of calorically dense items in each snack.** Try a two-item snack instead of three. Change one of the items to a fruit or vegetable to reduce the caloric density of these snacks.

- **Try the "33-33-33 percent plate" instead of the standard "50-25-25 percent plate."**

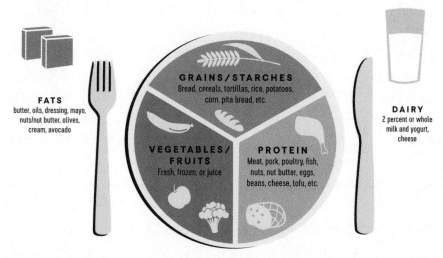

FATS
butter, oils, dressing, mayo,
nuts/nut butter, olives,
cream, avocado

GRAINS/STARCHES
Bread, cereals, tortillas, rice, potatoes,
corn, pita bread, etc.

VEGETABLES/
FRUITS
Fresh, frozen, or juice

PROTEIN
Meat, pork, poultry, fish,
nuts, nut butter, eggs,
beans, cheese, tofu, etc.

DAIRY
2 percent or whole
milk and yogurt,
cheese

This plate will increase the proportion of fruits and vegetables as well as the protein content while reducing the grains/starches. Grains and starches are an energy-rich food group that is easily digestible and does not increase satiety. On the other hand, proteins and veggies do increase satiety, so your child will most likely not feel an increase in hunger if the proportions at their meals change from the standard 50-25-25 percent plate to the 33-33-33 percent plate.

Increasing Your Child's Independence

Once your child is weight-restored, as well as medically and psychologically stable, you may begin to involve them in food choices. At this point, your child most likely has not chosen, plated, planned, or cooked a meal in months. However, in order to "return to normal" (see chapter 15) your child will need to be incrementally involved once more.

One of the first steps in this process is to allow your child to plate their meal. You should continue to prepare the meal and your child can plate it on their own. It's a "safe" experiment in that we ask you to approve the plate and adjust it as necessary if your child struggles to plate an acceptable amount of food. This will help your child reconnect with food, as they think about, touch, and plate food once again. If plating goes well, your child can begin to pack their school lunches, with your sign-off.

Or, you may ask your child to "choose a snack on their own." Again, this is safe, in that you continue to approve and adjust as necessary to meet your child's nutritional needs. This task will give you insight into how committed your child is to their recovery. Can they think of appropriate snacks and plate enough volume? If your child chooses grapes and carrot sticks as their snack, they probably aren't ready for this step.

These choices really characterize how strong or weak the eating disorder is and can provide valuable data about your child's readiness for increased freedom and decreased structure. Your child will need to choose an adequate variety and volume of food at meals and snacks, and they will need to continue to incorporate challenging foods, as they are already accustomed to eating at this stage.

Last, if things are going well, you can begin to test whether your child can eat lunch independently at school. Combined with medical monitoring, you will know pretty quickly if something is wrong. If your child loses weight during this time, they likely need increased supervision. But if your child is successful, it will increase confidence around food between you and your child, which sets the stage for a complete return to "normal eating" in the future.

Discuss whether your child is ready for "intuitive eating."
One way to decrease the meal plan might be to allow your child to begin to listen to their own hunger and satiety cues. This intuitive approach to "normalize" eating will be discussed further in chapter 15, but it necessitates that your child is ready for this step. There are several criteria we look for to determine whether a child is ready: they are at their goal weight, getting regular periods, eating spontaneously, and successfully eating meals on their own. As your child prepares for weight maintenance, this might be a good time to explore whether this is appropriate for your child. If so, this step can be complicated, and we suggest carefully considering such a transition with the entire treatment team.

Case Example: Rose

At sixteen years old, Rose had lost approximately thirty pounds due to anorexia nervosa. She was hospitalized for low heart rate and blood pressure instabilities, as well as severe malnutrition (weight below 75 percent of expected body weight). Rose gained ten pounds during her hospital admission and then was referred to an outpatient FBT team.

Rose and her parents followed through with the FBT recommendations. However, Rose's eating-disorder behaviors were strong, and she fought every meal, refusing many, and

---

refusing liquid supplementation as well. She was pulled out of school and all activities, and her mother took a leave of absence from work in order to care for Rose at home. During this time, her parents supervised all meals and snacks, and were relentless in refeeding their daughter.

Rose's parents increased her meals and snacks throughout her treatment, provided strict supervision, and had the extra support they needed to help her gain the weight she needed to be healthy. At the point that Rose was nearly at her goal weight range, she had resumption of menses. The family then began to ask, how do we help her maintain this weight? The treatment team suggested that Rose reach the middle of her goal weight range, rather than stop at the very minimum acceptable weight. This would help provide a "buffer" should she get sick or relapse. At this point, all of Rose's eating-disorder behaviors had ceased. She was happy, calm, and both experimental and flexible with all foods in all food situations. Her parents agreed that Rose gaining the remaining few pounds, while perhaps not essential, would help them feel more confident in her strong medical and psychological stability. Beyond that, the treatment team continued to monitor her growth to ensure she remained on track.

CHAPTER 12

How to Talk About Diet and Weight (Hint: Don't!)

"My clothes don't fit anymore, why do I need to keep gaining weight?!"

"You don't eat snacks, why should I?"

"All of my friends are skinnier than me. This isn't fair!"

AMONG THE MANY tough questions your child will ask you during treatment, some of the toughest are about weight and diet. Your child's eating disorder creates an intense fear around eating, weight gain, and the need to exercise, which is so strong that rational discussions about "what your medical provider said" and "what your blood work shows" may not register.

As you may have noticed, kids with eating disorders become very focused on everyone else's plate, body size, and/or exercise patterns. Your child may start asking why their sister is allowed to leave food on her plate, or why you are going to the gym when they cannot. They may ask why their best friend only needs to have a sandwich at lunch while they need to have a sandwich plus chips and yogurt. Or they may tell you with precise detail how much their friends weigh, or who wants to lose weight. They will claim that it is unfair for anyone else in the house to eat less than them or to exercise when they are not allowed to. Your child (or rather their eating disorder) will want to hold all members of the family hostage around food, exercise, and weight. A good rule of thumb is for each family member to focus on their own needs, and when it comes to the topic of food, weight, and shape, to keep your comments private.

When asked about how to respond to a child's questions about their weight, Elizabeth Scott, LCSW and cofounder of the Body Positive suggests, "Let's find the weight at which your body really whirs. Then work on accepting that weight. It is not about a number on a scale. . . . It is when you feel best and you are healthy and your brain works. If that weight is above the social ideal, well then you will need to work on self-compassion and a fierce sense of self-protection."

Liana Rosenman, cofounder of Project HEAL (a nonprofit that funds the treatment of eating disorders for those in need), encourages kids to "redefine what you think is beautiful. . . . It really has nothing to do with how someone looks. Find someone you think is beautiful and ask yourself why you think they are beautiful? Most of the things you say about them probably have nothing to do with physical beauty but actually their character, confidence etc. I find those who give back and help others to be beautiful." She recalls struggling herself with her body as she gained weight during her own recovery from her eating disorder but eventually came to realize that her body was capable of doing amazing things. "I wasn't going to be able to do the things I wanted if I was damaging my body—which was more of my vehicle to get where I wanted to get in my life." To get through it, she used the mantra "feeling is healing" and told herself that once she overcame *these* hard feelings, she could overcome anything.

Your child's concerns and fears about their weight/body are rooted in their worries about what the future of recovery looks like: "What if I gain a million pounds?" or "What if I look fat when this is over?" It's best to refocus your child to the present moment. We recommend the child take ten deep breaths, and sometimes even prescribe ten deep breaths prior to and after meals to help calm the body and mind. It's hard to think about "gaining weight" while concentrating on deep breathing.

Treat your child's distress like any other time your child was upset. Hold their hand and tell them that you are here for them and love them. And because you love them so much, you will not allow the eating disorder to take over. The what-if scenarios can be endless and highly anxiety provoking. It's best to try to encourage your child to avoid going down that road. You might tell them that the goal is for them to be healthy and safe, and while there are tons of possibilities about "what if," you want them to worry about what they have to do right now (which usually means: eat).

Working with your therapist to have accessible tools available in these emotional moments is very helpful to manage anxiety and other emotions that may come up like sadness, frustration, or anger. Distraction activities are used to help your child stay present versus hanging out in the future pondering hypothetical situations. Ideas for distraction activities are covered in chapter 14, but some examples include: painting, drawing, watching a movie, taking a shower, going for a walk (if cleared), playing a game, or chatting with a friend on the phone.

All Food Is Good Food

While your child needs to gain weight, you may not need to, or maybe you've even already experienced some weight gain as an unwanted side effect of caring for your child with an eating disorder. You might be saying to yourself, "My cholesterol is sky-high and I'm twenty pounds overweight—there are certain things I just can't eat. How do I manage that while having a child with anorexia?" Parents often have their own nutritional needs that may pose a direct conflict with their child's needs. For example, a parent may have been told that he or she is prediabetic and must avoid large portions of carbohydrates and added sugars. Or perhaps a parent is on a low-fat/low-sodium diet for heart disease. A parent may even have their own history of an eating disorder and may struggle with their own food fears.

Each family member is entitled to his or her own meal plan and approach to diet and nutrition. However, talking about diets, dieting, and "bad" foods in front of your child is not advised under any circumstances, as these might trigger your child's eating disorder. Talking about "cutting carbs" or "avoiding saturated fats" could make your child feel bad about eating what's on their plate. Comments about wanting to avoid desserts is likely to make your child feel guilty about eating those foods, reinforcing the notion that there are "bad foods" out there. Hearing a parent say that "they aren't going to eat much at dinner because they ate *way too much* at lunch" teaches a child to intellectually adjust their diet, rather than letting their body naturally decide, which is something they will need to learn how to do down the road. These types of comments make it even harder than it already is to eat. A better approach is to have your family adopt an "all food is good food" mentality at home and work together to model balanced eating.

Resist the Urge to "Weigh In"

In the early phases of treatment, when your child is truly struggling, it's better to avoid weight conversation altogether. Talking about weight in any way can be potentially volatile. Innocent comments may cause your child to restrict or change their diet, or turn to a negative coping mechanism. This may feel like avoidance, but it's truly better to say nothing and to instead remind your child that you love and care for them, than to say something seemingly harmless that sets them off. Discussions about weight, especially in the early stages of treatment, are an uphill battle, one that you will never win.

There will come a time when your child *can* hear about their weight, talk about their weight, and even talk about your weight in a healthy and normal way. However, now is not that time. At this point, talking about weight reminds your child about their wish to weigh less. Any comments about weight or shape, even those that you think are positive and helpful, are actually quite harmful to your child. Your child may interpret your seemingly benign comment "You look so much better than you used to look when you were sick" as "Oh, so I'm fat now?!" This is a very real example that showcases just how far an eating disorder can skew your words. Instead, when complimenting your child, it's best to take the focus off weight by saying, "Your personality is back" or "You seem so much more energetic now."

Similarly, parents should avoid commenting on other people's bodies. "She looks good," can be interpreted as "I should lose weight so I look good." Hearing about your friend's recent weight loss and "how great they look" reinforces that being thin is valued. Making a comment that Aunt Sally "got so much bigger" than when you saw her last time highlights that you notice these changes, and disapprove of them. This will terrify your child, and cause them to worry: "What if I get bigger, what will my parents and the rest of the world think of me then?"

It's inevitable that just as you are beginning to feel more confident in the fight against your child's eating disorder, you may go to a family function with your extended family, and find your aunt Ramona chatting in the corner about how she lost thirty-five pounds by cutting out carbohydrates, white flour, and sugars. This can be unsettling for your child, and confusing, as your child is seeking to reestablish their relationship with food. They may wonder if they, too, should avoid these foods, or it may reinforce that something is wrong with these foods. This will undoubtedly make family outings stressful and dreaded by you and your child.

If this happens, it can be helpful to pull your family member aside privately and explain that you have a no-weight-talk rule in the house to support your child struggling with an eating disorder. Share with your family member what's going on for your child, and why what they said was difficult for your child to hear. They should understand. According to Elizabeth Scott, "It is important to explore with your relative what messages they have received about their own bodies and how those messages made *them* feel. Explore with your child how they feel when they hear these messages from family members. Empower your child to address how they feel in family therapy. Advocate for your child and stop the relative with your authority to back up your child. If that is all they get out of treatment, being able to set limits on destructive messages projected at them, well that is a worthy treatment."

Remember, you don't have to go it alone. Your treatment team will also be teaching your child strategies to field these messages about food, weight, and shape. And while you will work to create an oasis of safety for your child, especially during recovery, the reality is that someone, somewhere will be talking about their new diet, or their desire to lose weight. It is imperative that you and the team work on building your child's armor so that these comments don't shake them as much. This can be accomplished by refocusing your child on "what's healthy for them?" For them to be healthy, they need to gain weight and eat a balanced plate that contains all food groups. Most kids know that being fearful of foods, and avoidant of food categories entirely, does not represent normal, fearless eating. They will need to be constantly reminded of this.

Modeling a Healthy Approach to Food

Inevitably, as your child struggles to eat, you may also be struggling with how to eat in front of your child. Some parents "power-eat"—eating larger than normal meals—to emphasize that there's nothing wrong with eating a lot. But the reality is, you might also feel frustrated that you have gained weight in the process of nourishing your child. Your sympathy for what your child is going through is palpable, and perhaps you have been eating what they eat, when they eat, in full support of their recovery process. However, this means you have not been listening to your own needs.

It is possible to support and sympathize with what your child is going through, and to take care of your own needs at the same time. Assess your current food intake: how does it differ from what you were eating before your child was diagnosed with an eating disorder? The most important things are that your child sees you eating regularly, eating a variety of foods, and eating flexibly. If this is something you cannot do due to an active eating disorder of your own or other food struggles, it can be effective to share this with your child in a family therapy session. Some parents may deny that there is a problem or may try to defend their eating patterns. However, if you exhibit any disordered or abnormal eating, it sends a confusing message to your child about what healthy should be. Scott suggests, "Since dieting is a powerful risk factor for the development (and maintenance) of an eating disorder, to consider dieting in front of a child with an eating disorder can be a lot like drinking in front of a family member in alcoholic rehab. Don't do it! Show support by accepting your own body. Get help with your body image issues."

Here are some tips for meeting your needs while modeling food flexibility for your child:

- **Eat three meals per day, minimum.** If your child sees you skip a meal, they will learn that food restriction is okay. This is also generally recommended for health in all individuals.
- **Eat a wide variety of food groups.** You can use the Plate-by-Plate approach for yourself as well, adjusting the proportions of foods to meet your own needs. You may need 25 to 33 percent grains/starch or a smaller portion of protein and a larger portion of vegetables.
- **Include fats.** There is a growing body of research about the benefits of eating fats (especially oils, nuts, and other plant-based fats). Please don't ever let your child see you eating a dry salad—that tends to send the message to your child that fats are "bad."
- **Eat at least one snack per day with your child.** Maybe that's dessert in the evening or a banana midmorning, either way, your child will begin to understand that you are following your own hunger cues and that it's okay and very normal to eat between meals.
- **Go out to dinner and *enjoy* your food!** Talk about the colors and flavors on your plate. Explain how fun it is to eat out because it allows you to try something new and different. Show your child that it's okay to eat a piece of bread with butter or chips and salsa before the main entrée comes. Show them how you eat some but not all of that basket of goodies so that you can enjoy your meal, too. In doing this you are modeling normal eating.

- **Explain your needs.** For example, if you have a specific diet that you need to follow due to medical complications, let your child know that just as you are helping them follow a specific meal plan to meet their needs, you also are following your own, and both of you are doing it to better your health. Let them know you have nutritional differences based on your own individual needs, and that's okay.

How to Handle Exercise

In the early phases of treatment your child won't be allowed to exercise at all, but you shouldn't have to stop being active. What's most important is that your child sees that you engage in activity because it makes you feel good, not because you need to lose weight. If possible, find time for exercise when your child is out of the house, at school, or with friends. It will be important for you and your spouse to take turns; you head to the gym while your spouse is spending time with your child. You don't need to exercise in secret, but you do need to be mindful of how your child will feel when you exercise and they cannot.

The same goes for activities and sports in which your other children are involved. While you may not be able to avoid taking your child with an eating disorder to their sibling's soccer game, look for alternatives wherever possible. Perhaps they can spend time with the neighbors while you go to your other child's game. It is also important for you to have open and honest discussions with your child about why you engage in activity. Explain that it decreases stress and increases serotonin, the "feel good" hormone. Let them know that moderate physical activity is a part of your daily life and that in order to have energy for exercise you eat regular meals and snacks and stay hydrated. Let them know your exercise is fun and enjoyable and not an obligation. If, as you're reading this, you are realizing that your exercise isn't fun or enjoyable, it may be time for *you* to rethink your activity as well! This is a time of reflection and growth for the entire family. Helping a child through recovery will open your eyes to what "health" means for all of you.

Facing Your Fears

As your child nears their goal weight range, you may find yourself growing anxious because your child is nearing the weight they were at when this all started, and the thought of them spiraling downward again because of their unhappiness with that weight is terrifying. Some parents even worry that their child is "bigger" than they've ever been. Often, parents seem to be on board with weight gain until they see their child physically gaining weight, then they start questioning the need for further weight gain. You may find yourself thinking, "Are those last five pounds really necessary?" According to Scott, "This is the time to address your beliefs and feelings that underlie those concerns about weight gain." She writes:

> You will want to explore the feelings and content you associate with weight. Given the culture families live in today, messages about fat are often tangled with power, access, and success. In the process, you may uncover fears that your child will be stigmatized if they become fat or that they will lose the privileges associated with slenderness in this society. It is useful to identify these fears and to learn to see how pressuring your child to be thin is not unlike pressuring them to be whiter, it might bring privilege but if it is not your child's natural weight/race then the cost is too high. It is better

to teach your child to defend their body from criticism as you would confront racism if your child is black or brown skinned.

When treating a child with an eating disorder, at first it may seem like they are the sole focus and the treatment is entirely for them. However, most parents learn a lot about their own food and weight biases along the way. This is a time to also work on your own relationship with food and weight in order to truly support your child. You are not alone in this struggle and there are great resources out there to help you *and* your child reestablish a healthy relationship with food. For additional resources see page 273.

CHAPTER 13

Eating
on the Road

THE **PLATE-BY-PLATE APPROACH** is applicable to all settings, across all types of cuisine. Eating out is your child's ticket to freedom. Being okay with food from outside the house is an important part of your child's social life and allows them to go to restaurants, friends' houses, parties, and barbecues; participate in holidays; and, eventually, go off to college. Eating out helps to challenge aspects of your child's eating disorder and teaches them to eat what's served, order from menus, and let go of the demand to always know how the food is prepared. This inevitably helps to cultivate flexibility, but it will take a lot of practice for your child to master eating outside of their home environment. In this chapter and the next, Chapter 14: Moving Beyond Brown Rice, you'll find strategies to teach your child the skills associated with eating out, all in the spirit of helping your child to become a fearless and confident eater.

Eating outside of the home is challenging for kids with eating disorders. Decoding menus and restaurant cooking/portions, adjusting to altered meal schedules, and calculating different time zones associated with travel are just some of the challenges that a child with an eating disorder might face. Some children report feeling overwhelmed, while others are in a state of panic looking at all of the options on the menu and trying to choose the best meal. They could read the menu for hours, if allowed. They describe their fears about the way in which the food may be prepared (Does the chef add oils? butter?) and worry about how big the serving will be. International cuisines might be daunting. Navigating these obstacles during the early stages of an eating disorder will be more of a struggle than in the later stages when the eating disorder has quieted. Later in recovery your child will become more flexible and intuitive with their eating, though these obstacles will remain a challenge. If you are not sure how your child will tolerate meal outings, going out can provide you with insight into your child's eating disorder. By experimenting, you'll find out how they handle themselves and what skills you both already possess, or need to further hone, in order to manage eating-disorder behaviors at a restaurant.

Your child might eventually express that they are interested and ready to eat out. Whoa! Is that possible? you ask. It can and will happen as your child gets further along in recovery. Practice has to start somewhere, and you will never know how the experience will actually go until you try. In the depths of the illness, your child will most likely want to run in the other direction from a restaurant, wishing to avoid eating out altogether. They will be anxious at the mere mention of it. When the time is right, however, your child will need to be pushed by you and by the treatment team to take the Plate-by-Plate approach on the road.

So how do you know when to allow your child to go out to eat? There is no exact recipe or formula for making this decision. Like most aspects of this process, you'll need to rely on your instincts.

Your child may be ready for this step if they are mostly compliant with meals at home, without pushback, though this isn't a requirement. If your child has met medical milestones such as reaching their goal weight range, having improved vital signs, or resuming menses, the eating disorder is likely getting quieter. Typically, the more weight restored and nourished a child is, the quieter their eating disorder becomes. As a child reaches their goal weight range, we tend to see increased flexibility and acceptance of food. Being in a good place medically, while also seeming ready psychologically, is another good sign that it's time for you to test the waters out of the house.

As you consider whether to travel or eat in restaurants, you will need confidence that you've got this and that you can apply the Plate-by-Plate approach. If your child will only eat "this one kind of bread" and only boneless skinless chicken breast that is dry without any sauce, they likely are not ready to eat in a restaurant. A restaurant requires flexibility and will quickly test your child's eating disorder. However, if they have practiced eating your chicken Parmesan at home, and you both have found it to be a successful meal, then next time you're in the mood for it go to your local Italian restaurant instead. By trying more challenging meals at home first, you and your child are practicing the skills necessary to be successful on the road.

Supervised Meals (Phase 1 FBT)

Meal excursions can occur when you are in charge of all meals (Phase 1 FBT) or when your child is becoming more independent (Phases 2 and 3), or both. Outings that occur during Phase 1 can be more difficult and strained. Ordering, eating, and finishing the meal would likely be a struggle. Being in public adds an additional challenge, as it becomes tempting to give in to the eating disorder in public settings—for example, by allowing your child to order a salad because you know they will finish it, or allowing them to not finish the plate because you can't realistically stay at the restaurant table for as long as you would need to. The pressure of being in public might make you feel that your power is limited. However, as the parent in charge, you can decide what you feel is best for your child in that moment. Know that you can always pick up the plan when you return home. Restaurants are tough for someone in the early stages of an eating disorder but get much easier as the eating disorder gets quieter. A child in Phase 1 cannot sufficiently decide what or how much to eat, often getting stuck on how many calories or fat grams any one dish may contain. It can be stressful for your child as an inner conflict emerges between getting what looks good and what might be the "healthier" option. In this stage, if your child was in charge of ordering, they may drive the waiter nuts to meet the needs of their eating disorder: "I'll have the turkey club sandwich, on sliced wheat bread, no aioli, no bacon, no cheese, no avocado, and can you please substitute a side salad for the french fries, hold the dressing?" If your child were allowed to choose their meal, they would likely become highly distressed and anxious.

And under those circumstances, the odds are against them in succeeding to order a nutritionally adequate meal, so parents should expect to take over all aspects of restaurant ordering on behalf of their child.

During Phase 1 of FBT, where presumably your child is more medically fragile, meal outings will be tough and might not be the best idea. If you must go, the priority is that your child has a sufficient balance and volume of food at the meal. We have worked with families who felt scared to take their child out to eat and settled on letting their child order "just a salad." "At least they ate!" the parents say. They were happy that the child ordered from the menu at all . . . and ate what they ordered! Unfortunately, this outcome would allow your child's eating disorder to thrive. Practice makes perfect, and this will take practice.

You may be wondering how just one nutritionally inadequate meal could matter that much. Here's the thing: even if your child has graduated from the medical danger zone, they are still recovering. Think about it—would you allow your wheelchair-bound child with a broken leg to get up for five minutes because they are angry and frustrated at their lack of mobility? Maybe they'll be strong enough to avoid any real risk, and it is easier to say yes than no when your child is miserable, but this puts them at risk for damaging their leg further. If your child is allowed to eat plain salad at a restaurant for one meal just to make them "feel better," the eating disorder thrives and your child remains sick. And in some cases, that one inadequate meal can cause your child to take a few steps back in their recovery. You are being tasked with the crucial art of remaining steadfast in the face of the eating disorder. It's not easy, we know. But by not wavering, you are showing your child that you've got this on their behalf, even if they are actively struggling.

Allowing the eating disorder to sit at the table, even for one meal, can send a message to your child that the eating disorder is allowed to manipulate mealtime again. It can cause you and your child to lose your footing and it is risky. It will also very likely cause the next nutritionally complete meal to cause feelings of guilt and frustration, as your child resumes following the Plate-by-Plate approach. Phase 1 of FBT is a time of acute healing.

Similar to a period during which someone is undergoing surgical rehabilitation, kids with eating disorders are expected to lay low and heal, and your job is to help protect your child's recovery at all costs.

Unsupervised Meals (Phases 2 and 3 FBT)

Unsupervised meals happen either because the child is ready for this next step, or because there is a can't-miss event that comes up. Either way, when your child is choosing and eating an unsupervised meal on their own, they should plan to eat more than they think they need. Unfortunately, it is much more common for a child with an eating disorder to greatly under-shoot the mark, assuming for example that restaurant meals are inherently "heavier." This is a good reason for your child to stick to the Plate-by-Plate approach, which can easily be followed while out of the house. They should run through whether all food groups are present, whether the plate is full, whether it's plated in the right ratios, and aim to finish most of the plate.

When There's a Must-Attend Event

We have heard about thousands of these events through our clients' stories—whether it's the end-of-the-year dance recital, auditions for the school play, or a once-in-a-lifetime tour of their favorite baseball team's clubhouse. We would much prefer your child be ready for an unsupervised event, but realistically, that's not the order in which this is most likely to occur. What to do?

First, if your child is really struggling, we urge you to strongly consider having your child sit out from the event. As with eating out at restaurants, if your child isn't ready or will not be supervised by you during this event, it can set them up for failure. Attending an event, even one where only one or two meals might be affected, can cause your child to backtrack and increase their anxiety and distress. Despite the can't-miss event, we ask you to separate out the emotions around the event and make a decision that is best for your child's recovery.

If your child must attend the event and you don't think they are ready to eat an unsupervised meal, you should consider a strategy to maximize the food your child is consuming in front of you, while minimizing the amount of food your child is eating away from you. For example, if the event means your child will not be with you at lunch, then you can send your child with part of their lunch, such as a sandwich and fruit, but then have them eat a larger snack when they get home. Alternatively, you can consider having your child eat an early lunch prior to the event. This will ensure they complete all meals and snacks with you. And although they will have to tolerate an altered meal schedule, if the event is important enough to them, they will likely be motivated to complete their meals anyway. Making a game plan for these instances will help to keep your child on track with their nutrition, while minimizing the risk associated with unsupervised meals.

When Your Child Is Ready for Less Supervision

As your child progresses in recovery, more independence around food is a natural next step and can give insight into the stage of your child's eating disorder. As you progress from the intense supervision of Phase 1, it is normal to feel nervous about entering the next phase. Can you trust that your child's eating disorder has receded enough such that they can plate their own meal properly and eat everything? This is a pivotal moment. After all of this hard work you pull back slightly to see how firm a hold the eating disorder has or does not have over your child.

Eating one meal away from the family is a relatively safe experiment. Once in phases 2 and 3 of FBT, they are not as fragile and not as susceptible to ups and downs. At this point, they have proven to you that they are capable of completing their meals without a fight and they are more committed to their recovery than in Phase 1. With close medical monitoring, you will be able to assess whether the child was able to succeed while on their own. Their weight will likely start to trend downward or their vital signs will worsen if they are secretly throwing away part of their lunch at school. If your child has a history of purging, you may see that their urine pH becomes elevated if they begin purging again. These are reasons why parents should test their child with only one or two unsupervised meals per week, so if it isn't going well, the child doesn't deteriorate quickly. Here baby steps are key. Knowing whether your child's eating disorder is quiet enough to allow for success with unsupervised meals can help you make future decisions about autonomy more easily. If they are successful, additional unsupervised meals can be added.

Things to Consider

As you begin to consider allowing an unsupervised meal, you should first assess how *you* feel about it:

- Is your child compliant with meals at home when you aren't around?
- Do you think your child will succeed?
- Do you think your child is ready for this challenge?
- Does this challenge come at a good time in your child's life? Food experiments, if carried out during a stressful time like final exams or during a family move, are less likely to be successful.

We know you will feel anxious about this step, but what does your instinct tell you? This is similar to that feeling when your child first learned how to ride a bike: that moment of letting go and trusting that if they fall, their knee pads and helmet will protect them. Your child has learned many skills along this journey and has found motivation for recovery. And while "falls" are still going to happen, your child is protected from falling too hard because they have practiced over and over again under your guidance.

It also is important to check in with your child about their readiness to eat an unsupervised meal:

- How does your child feel about completing a meal without a parent supervising?
- Does your child really want to go to their friend's birthday party— pizza *and* cake without you there to help them through it?
- Are they scared?
- Do they, themselves, feel they know their nutritional needs well enough to succeed?

You would expect your teenager to be begging to go out with their friends, but anxiety about "getting it right" is common and your child has every right to be scared. Remind them that you are confident in their ability to face their fears and to ask for help when they need it. Instill confidence in your child that they can do this and that you'll be there if they do "fall."

Eating disorders take a huge emotional, physical, and financial toll on everyone in the family. You and your child will not want to backtrack as you recall the challenges of Phase 1 while they were gaining weight, how restricted their life was, how sad they felt, and how many doctors' appointments they had. As you and your child enter Phase 2 and then 3 of FBT, you have had a taste for what life can look and feel like in the absence of the eating disorder. This may cause your child to want to protect their recovery much more than before. As clinicians, we are always amazed at the honesty our clients express when we ask them about their fears about gaining food autonomy. They might say, "I am nervous about getting distracted at the concert and not being able to eat my snack." Or "I am worried about eating in front of so many people and whether or not they'll judge my larger meals."

Case Example: Hugo

Hugo had a full-day writers' workshop to attend that would require him to eat lunch and one snack on his own. He was medically stable and doing well enough that his parents wanted to let him try. When his parents checked in with him ahead of time, Hugo shared that he was worried that no one else would be eating when he had to, and he felt intimidated to eat in front of his peers. He and his parents discussed meeting in the school parking lot for those meals so he could come out of the workshop to eat under supervision and then return. Ultimately, Hugo realized he was mostly worried that his eating would be too loud, and would be a big distraction to the classroom. So he and his parents collaboratively decided that he could choose "quiet" foods such as yogurt, walnuts, and cantaloupe for snack, and a PB&J sandwich, cheese slices, and grapes for lunch; all of which would be less noisy, and therefore less embarrassing to eat during the workshop.

Talking through your child's specific concerns is a great way for you to work with your child, as a team, to troubleshoot and think through the upcoming event. This helps your child succeed while building their confidence about how to accomplish their meal.

It would also be wise to set up some way to hold your child accountable for the meal. You can ask them to send a photo of their unsupervised meal via text, perhaps even a before and after shot. Or, if that's too "weird" while they're out with their friends, ask them to report back to you when they get home. After your child completes the unsupervised meal, whether they were deemed ready or not, it is advisable for you to check in with your child afterward. How did it go? Did they eat 100 percent of the plate? What did they have? This helps to hold your child accountable and will make them feel more supported in this experiment. If given too much freedom, the eating disorder could creep back in, making an unsupervised meal an opportunity to eat less. If your child was unable to eat 100 percent of what they were supposed to have, you can give your child an added snack to make up for whatever was missed, and then let them know you appreciate their honesty and commitment to recovery.

Is Your Child Ready for Unsupervised Meal Outings?

- Nearing or has reached goal weight range
- Medically stable
- Resumption of menses
- Compliant with supervised meal and snacks

- Flexible with food
- Seems up for the experiment
- Committed to recovery

You should ask yourself:

- Has my child's eating disorder receded enough to allow them to succeed at unsupervised meals?
- Does my child demonstrate a good understanding of the meal plan in order to easily plate an appropriate meal?
- Do I think my child will succeed?
- Do I think my child is ready for this challenge?
- What is my gut reaction to whether my child is ready for this step?

Check in with your child and ask:

- Do you really want to go?
- Are you scared?
- Do you feel you know the Plate-by-Plate approach well enough to succeed?
- Do you have any specific concerns?
- Do you need any additional guidance about planning for the event?

Eating in Restaurants

Be warned: If home-cooked meals and food in general are scary for your child, your child may consider restaurants and buffets a nightmare. Prepare for this to be a challenge for any child suffering from an eating disorder. Restaurants serve large portions, often list calories on the menu, and the meals are full of unknown ingredients. Your child will translate all of that into meaning "extra calories, fat, and weight gain." We have had kids show up to restaurants with measuring cups and food scales in tow, a sign the child is clearly not ready to enter the world of restaurant eating.

Given that eating out will be difficult for your child, you will first want to choose a meal that will foster success in this setting. Even if the meal feels overly "safe," such as chicken, broccoli, and rice, it will still be challenging for your child because it is being prepared at a restaurant. As the child gets more comfortable eating out, you can increase the challenge level of the meal.

As you navigate different types of restaurant meals, ask yourself, are all food groups present and is it enough? A worksheet can be found on page 209 where you can map out what food groups are present at a variety of meals on the road. The priority when eating out is to make sure the plate is adequate, and when restaurants don't have certain food items, it is important to add extras (whatever food group you want) to cover for the volume expected on that plate. For example, when going to Japanese or Chinese restaurants, it might be difficult to add a dairy item. In that case, you can add a different drink instead (juice or soda), or else add an extra item onto your child's plate, such as an egg roll or edamame.

Due to the fact that restaurant portions can be large, we ask that you use your judgment in deciding how much your child needs to eat. It might mean that you ask your child to consume only 75 percent of the plate, depending on how large the plate is. But you can decide what seems right, and aim to follow the Plate-by-Plate approach as best as you can, aiming for a plate that is full, and contains starch, protein, vegetables, fats, and dairy.

If your child is participating in an unsupervised meal outing on their own, they should also plan to eat at least 75 percent of their plate to ensure nutritional adequacy. For these outings to be successful, your child should be in touch with reality around food portions. They should be able to determine if the portion served is really large or whether they just perceive it to be large. They should have a sense of how to gauge how much they need (more or less) and be able to stick to it. And lastly, they should be honest about the process. Can they admit the areas in which they struggled? Kids who are committed to recovery may share a misstep with their parents (rather than hiding it) and be able to add more to another meal/snack to make up for missed food.

Being able to accept food as it arrives—and seeing that nothing bad happened as a result of experiencing the unknown—allows kids to become fearless and confident eaters. Those are helpful skills to have when traveling, going to college, or going out with friends on a day trip.

Practicing eating out once per week (or whatever your family's budget may afford) is usually a good idea, in the spirit of recovery. Some families may say, "We don't eat out much because we are on a strict budget." It's understandable, however this can also be considered an "investment" in your child's future food freedom. Eating out provides a unique opportunity to see what comes up for your child, if anything. Avoiding restaurants as a family might convey to your child that "something is wrong with eating out." If you never ordered take-out for dinner, or never went to a restaurant, you would never know how your child would respond in these settings. Eating out also doesn't have to be expensive; it could be fast food or a sandwich from the grocery-store deli counter, the most important thing is that your child is exposed to food that is not cooked at home.

Case Example: Dasha

Dasha's family did a lot of home cooking and rarely ate in restaurants, but her friends liked to go out to eat. When she went out with a friend's family and they decided they would stop by Chipotle for lunch, she began to feel sweaty, dizzy, and anxious. She was surprised about this reaction, as she had been in the late stages of recovery from her eating disorder for a long time already. However, her anxiety grew as she neared the restaurant. She was unable to recover from the anxiety that flooded her, and she eventually asked to go home.

As parents, you want to know whether your child can successfully navigate a restaurant and you will need to find out whether the restaurant environment increases their anxiety. Are certain cuisines more stressful than others? Can your child order easily and swiftly from a menu? How do they handle the portion sizes that are served in restaurants?

Restaurant Planning Worksheet

Use this table to help track which types of restaurants your child has tried. The food group columns will help you think through the meal to create a balanced plate.

	GRAINS/ STARCHES	PROTEIN	FRUIT/ VEGETABLES	FATS	DAIRY
BURGERS					
CHINESE					
DELI					
GERMAN					
GREEK					
INDIAN					
ITALIAN					
JAPANESE					
KOREAN					
MEXICAN					
THAI					

Buffets

Buffets can often be especially intimidating. There is usually an over-whelming amount of food, with several different types of foods served. If you are plating your child's meals, we suggest that your child sit at the table while you go up to the buffet and choose what to put on their plate. Otherwise, you will hear a lot of chatter about what your child wants and doesn't want. Listening to your child's demands appeases their eating disorder, rather than fights it. Expecting your child to sit at the table while you plate will empower you to provide your child with an adequate meal in an otherwise challenging setting.

For kids who are ready to be more independent with meals, a buffet can mimic a college dining hall setting and is a good place to practice making good plates. As our patients are heading off to college, we usually have them practice buffet dining at two or three different places. We suggest you start this "training" three or four months before they leave, to allow for enough trial and error for your child to gain the confidence needed to successfully eat in an otherwise challenging setting.

Travel

Typically, family travel is not recommended while your child is still struggling with strong eating-disorder behaviors. Travel tends to be difficult for both the parents and the child. For the child, travel brings challenges such as limited food options on a long car or plane ride, new foods, new ways of food preparation, different time zones, and an altered meal schedule—all of which can be hard for a child actively struggling with an eating disorder. In addition, going sightseeing can bump up the child's energy requirements, making the need for *even more* food essential. For you, it will be harder to stay on top of all of the meals while away, and it can be difficult to supervise your child. You may struggle to "fight the fight" while on the airplane, at restaurants, or in museums.

It goes without saying that if your child is medically fragile, it is not a good idea to travel. There is often very little room for error, and your child will likely need close medical monitoring, which often isn't possible while away. Families may end up canceling a vacation they planned many months in advance, or cut vacation short due to a child struggling with an eating disorder. While it's disappointing, most do not regret these decisions because it means their child is safe and taken care of. Your child can go from being medically fragile to medically unstable while away, making travel dangerous. We have had families need to check in with local doctors, who often aren't trained in eating-disorder management, or seek out hospitals. This certainly causes a lot of stress during what was supposed to be a relaxing family trip. If you must travel with your child while in the early stages of eating-disorder treatment, it may be safer to start with a shorter trip that is not too far from home.

But if your child is medically stable, you should assess whether you and your child can navigate the demands of travel. And if you are unsure, we suggest discussing it with your child's treatment team several months in advance. For a recovery-minded child, going away can serve as a good motivator. For example, Lorena wanted desperately to go on the upcoming ski trip with her cousins. For several weeks prior to the scheduled vacation, Lorena met every weight goal and was following her meal plan perfectly. She was more motivated than ever because she wanted to go on that trip. However, for another child, a trip of this nature could be too overwhelming, and frankly, too risky.

If traveling is deemed to be a good idea, and your child seems ready, we suggest that you plan on packing some of your child's favorite snacks as backup. The travel day alone can be arduous, with unexpected obstacles like canceled flights and long layovers. Being prepared can help your child stay on track. It can be helpful to pack some supplements, such as Ensure Plus or BOOST Plus, just in case you need to add to a suboptimal meal, or to make up for anything that might have been skipped or missed. Here's a handy list of nonperishable, portable snacks.

Easy Foods for Travel
- Nuts, trail mix
- Dried fruit: raisins, cranberries, mango, apricots

- Fresh fruit: apples, bananas, and oranges travel well
- Granola bars: pack one for each day. You might want to get higher- and lower-calorie bars for different situations. Higher-calorie bars include: PROBAR, Clif Builder's bar, Bounce bars. Lower-calorie bars include: KIND, LUNA, Chewy granola bars, fig bars, Nature Valley bars.
- Peanut butter, almond butter, cashew butter, or sunflower seed butter
- Beef jerky, turkey jerky
- Crunchy chickpeas
- Chips, pretzels, crackers
- Buttered popcorn
- Cookies, brownies
- Ensure/Boost Plus

Case Example: Sierra

Sierra, an eighteen-year-old female in recovery from her eating disorder, had spent the previous year in treatment. She was now eating independently, exercising a few times a week and feeling great. She struggled sometimes with including new foods, but for the most part, she was doing well and was planning to head off to college in the late summer. Then, her family took a trip to Hawaii. She did well with the food while there, navigated the buffets, and still kept up with her exercise classes. However, the resort was huge, and there was a lot of walking. And at night, the family often walked to dinner, which could be over a mile each way. This was a lot more activity than Sierra was used to, yet despite this increase in activity, she didn't increase her food intake and ultimately lost weight while on vacation.

This skill of adjusting how much one eats in different circumstances is essential for maintaining recovery in the real world, which can be unpredictable. Seeing this play out for Sierra gave her parents insight into an area of her eating disorder that was still alive. Without the trip, they wouldn't have seen this. This highlighted an area of recovery that still needed work: the ability to shift her food intake in response to changes in her environment. Her team asked her to adjust her exercise upward and downward, and then to rest, all while adjusting her food intake. She kept up with medical appointments to make sure her weight was stable as she tested her ability to adjust.

Frequently Asked Questions

Q: "I went out to a buffet with friends for my unsupervised meal. They had a lot of options, but the plates were small . . . definitely not ten inches. I wasn't sure what to do." —Child

A: Even for a child far along in recovery, a different plate size might make the meal difficult to navigate. In this case, the child should either plan to have several small plates, or aim for a "heaping plate of food."

Q: "My daughter went to a birthday party and had the cupcake but didn't eat the icing. I didn't make her eat more, because I figured it was great that she ate any of it! Is this okay?" —Parent

A: It's great your child was able to have some of the cupcake. This is an important step in normalizing your child's relationship with food. How did your child used to eat a cupcake? Did she used to eat the whole thing? If so, the goal is to get her back to "normal." If she used to eat all of the cupcake, we would ask you to provide another opportunity to practice eating a cupcake, and this time, ask your child to eat the whole thing. Practicing this over and over will help break down the fears associated with eating icing, and/or the whole cupcake.

Q: "I feel comfortable with my son eating lunch out with his friends on his own, but how often is too often?" —Parent

A: We recommend starting independent meal outings once or twice a week. If this proves successful, you can increase it from there. Remember, baby steps promote a sustainable recovery.

Eating on the road can pose challenges as well as present opportunities for growth. If you and your child have often been successful with meals at home, it is likely that your child is ready for a meal away. The key is to talk about it with your child and develop a game plan, which will allow you and your child to be successful in challenging situations. The more practice you have, the easier it will get.

CHAPTER 14

Moving Beyond
Brown Rice

Letting Go of Food Fears

"Introducing new foods is scary, but there comes a point when you realize how freeing it is to not be bound by rules, and that outweighs any scary and negative feeling associated with it. I had an entirely different concept of "healthy." I would go out of my way to make a pizza crust out of sweet potato and oats and convince myself it tasted better. And I almost felt above everyone else for it. But in reality, I was damaging my body and mind and it doesn't get anymore unhealthy than that. This is not to say that I don't still cringe at eating certain things, or over-analyze some foods, but that voice is slowly becoming quieter and my rational mind is able to win more often than not."
—Adolescent challenging her orthorexic food beliefs

"It took a long time for me to be able to see how debilitating orthorexia was and how it was just not a sustainable lifestyle. It seems so obvious and irrational from the outside, but the feeling is so powerful that when you're stuck that deep and you've convinced yourself for so long of your ways, it takes many "wake-up calls" to undo all the layers of denial."
—Adolescent working toward recovery from orthorexia

TEENS WHO MAINTAIN strict guidelines for what they will or will not eat are likely to continue being restrictive years later. To ensure a solid recovery, it is important to systematically work to improve your child's flexibility with a wide variety of foods. Ideally, recovery means eating birthday cake without fear, eating comfortably in restaurants or while traveling, and unwaveringly grabbing pizza with friends. In fact, we often tell our clients that learning how to eat pizza is mandatory in order to successfully go off to college. You are probably wondering how you will get from where you are currently to watching your child eat and actually *enjoy* pizza. But it is possible!

The day your child converts a food they feared to a food they once again embrace is an exciting milestone. Throughout this chapter, we will help you determine where your child's food vulnerabilities lie, and then how best to begin exposure, the process by which we ask you to reintroduce "fear foods" back into your child's diet.

True freedom from the grasp of the eating disorder is the primary goal, and this stage is a time for fine-tuning, to excavate remnants of eating-disorder thinking, and minimize distress, all while shaping your child into a confident and fearless eater. We want to see your teen get back to "normal," or rather what was normal for them *before* the onset of their eating disorder. Getting back to their normal usually means they are back to eating spontaneously and regularly throughout the day, with enjoyment, and with adequate variety.

4 Steps to Freeing Your Child from Their Food Fears

1. Identify what foods really push your child's buttons.
2. Commit to exposing your child to the food, and expect your child to finish it.
3. Don't ask your child if they want to try the food, decide for them.
4. Plan on repeated exposures to the food, done in several different circumstances.

What Are Your Child's Safe Foods? Fear Foods?

It is important for parents to have an understanding of which foods feel "safe" for their child and which are considered "fear foods." Safe foods are foods that your child thinks are easy to eat even when struggling with an eating disorder. Typically foods your child thinks are "good" or "healthy," your child does not have any fears associated with eating them and usually does not associate them with weight gain. Safe foods tend to be things such as vegetables, fruit, lean chicken, fish, and nonfat Greek yogurt. Sticking only to safe foods might mean your child is avoiding foods that contain sugar, carbohydrates, fats, or are processed snacks. The avoidance of these foods tends to reinforce their perceived fear. What are some of your child's safe foods?

Conversely, "fear foods" are foods that scare your child. Your child might think that a food is fattening or that eating it can cause immediate weight gain. They might label these foods "disgusting," "unhealthy," "gross," or "too high in sugar." Fear foods might include potato chips, ice cream, cookies, cake, brownies, and candy. Objectively, one food is not capable of "making someone fat." Too much of anything in excess of a person's requirements will cause weight gain, whether that is an excess of cookies or turkey or apples. We want your child to get a combination of safe foods, fear foods, and neutral foods (foods that are neither safe nor scary) in their diet. What are your child's fear foods?

To take the next step, we ask you to list your child's fear foods. Depending on where your child is at in recovery (still resisting treatment or willingly working toward it), you might be able to involve your child in this part. Can you create a food hierarchy? Choose which foods on that list would be the least scary and which would be the most. You and your child can rank this list, assigning a number value to indicate the least to most scary (0 = not scary at all, 10 = frightening!).

For example, parents Sarit and Dimitri and their son Zev made a list of Zev's fear foods:

- whole eggs
- white potatoes

- pizza
- pasta
- full-fat anything (yogurt, milk, cheese, sour cream, cream cheese)
- red meat
- all desserts (cookies, chocolate, candy, cakes, ice cream, milk shakes, etc.)
- farmed salmon (He prefers wild salmon.)
- mayonnaise
- salad dressing

Then we asked them to rank them on a scale of 0 to 10, with 10 being the "most scary."

- whole eggs: 3
- white potatoes: 6
- pizza: 6
- pasta: 5
- full-fat yogurt: 3
- red meat: 5
- all desserts (cookies, chocolate, candy, cakes, ice cream, milk shakes, etc.): 8
- farmed salmon: 2
- mayonnaise: 7
- salad dressing: 5

This exercise helped Sarit and Dimitri to notice which of the "fear foods" Zev was least scared of eating. It became clear to Sarit and Dimitri that salmon (ranked 2), whole eggs (3), and full-fat yogurt (3) were far less scary than desserts (8).

Food Exposure and the Importance of "Fighting the Fight"

Working on eradicating food fears takes courage and persistence. It takes a firm belief that this process will work, and it takes effort to fight against a resistant and unrelenting eating disorder. To rebuild your child's comfort level with certain foods, you will be asked to work on a technique psychologists call "exposure." Be aware that the process of exposure will escalate your child's anxiety, which will likely in turn make you anxious. There may be an increase in tears and arguing, yet all of that hard work is helping inch your child closer to the end goal of food freedom.

Exposure therapy typically is used to treat anxiety disorders, including panic disorder, certain phobias, and obsessive-compulsive disorder. Exposure works by confronting something that creates an escalation in anxiety and allowing a person, through repeated exposures of that trigger, to acclimate or "habituate" to it. This means that the more someone is exposed to something scary, the less fear they experience in its presence over time.

When sharing about exposure with one family, their son Jack enthusiastically said, "Mom, it's like the big red slide!" One summer at camp, Jack had been looking at "the big red slide," feeling too scared to go down. Instead, he spent his days watching his friends go down, screaming and laughing the whole way. Then one day, he mustered up the courage to just climb to the top of the ladder, and though nervous, decided to go down it. He loved it, and after that first time, he went on the slide over and over again, and didn't feel scared anymore.

As it relates to food, the fear of specific types of foods and methods of food preparation is a form of anxiety. Repeated exposures to a scary or avoided food allow your child to become desensitized to it over time. This allows them to eventually become comfortable, even if initially reluctant or avoidant. If your child can face their food fears, over time they will become used to it, while building positive experiences that reduce fear. The repeated aspect of the exposure is a learning process: instead of the food being attached to the belief that something bad will happen, the food becomes associated with the experience that all will be okay.

If your child maintains avoidance of foods, then it will only reinforce the negative thoughts and feelings around those foods. Avoidance prevents your child from getting the chance to experience (and thus learn) that they can tolerate food exposure.

Let's go back to Zev's list of "safe foods" and "fear foods." After his parents made the list, his mom, Sarit, decided to serve farmed salmon that very night, explaining to Zev that while wild salmon might offer some health advantages, he needs to be able to eat farmed salmon should he encounter that at a friend's house, or in a restaurant. Sarit said it confidently and didn't waver. She didn't ask him if that was okay (he would have absolutely said no!).

That night, Zev ate the farmed salmon. He said that while he didn't like it, it wasn't nearly as bad as he thought it would be. This gave Sarit and Zev the confidence to keep working through Zev's list of fear foods. They made an effort to repeat the exposures; they served farmed salmon several times (over several weeks), not just once. This allowed Zev to become desensitized to his fear. Sarit and Dimitri also worked on several other fear foods at the same time. They tackled full-fat yogurt and practiced having Zev eat several different brands and flavors. They served it in individual containers and out of a larger container, where portions were less defined. They sometimes added granola, berries, or used it in a smoothie.

When it came time to address Zev's fear of red meat, Sarit and Dimitri realized they needed to create a "hierarchy within a hierarchy" because the category of red meat felt so broad. They broke red meat down into subcategories and ranked Zev's fear of each one further: a burger was 5/10, ground taco meat was 6/10, a cheeseburger was 7/10, and steak was 8/10.

After brainstorming together, they decided they would first try a burger. These foods were harder for Zev. He asked his family to help distract him and take the focus away from the food that made him anxious. The family helped distract Zev by playing music in the background and discussing their favorite movies at the table. When he was done eating, they reminded him to take deep breaths. This type of work went on for months. As the family chipped away at Zev's food fears, they noticed the fears began to dissolve.

Zev was surprised to see that some foods weren't as scary as he had first thought. White potatoes, which he ranked as a 6, felt more like a 4 after he ate them. As you practice the exposures, keep track of the initial anxiety ratings; it is highly rewarding to watch as the anxiety ratings decrease after each exposure, and as foods are eventually crossed off the fear-foods list altogether.

Your child doesn't have to eat fear foods every day (but they certainly can!). It might be the case that while working on this area, your child may be eating several challenging foods a week. Some kids can handle adding one challenging item in daily, and others may need to work on this more slowly, trying two or three fear foods a week. Your child will best be able to identify the food areas that still push their buttons and increase their anxiety, assuming they are in a place of seeking a "true" recovery and are able to be open and honest. Admitting the areas that are still challenging helps your child chip away at—and eventually extinguish—any eating disorder thoughts that might be breathing below the surface. This helps to improve their relationship with food and can continue for years to come.

Set Challenges

Below is a list of "challenges" set by one of our clients. These challenges were foods that increased her anxiety. She created this list and systematically worked on eating each and every one of them, despite it being difficult for her. Try these with your kid, and have them set their own.

- Have real ice cream from an ice cream shop
- Eat a whole bagel
- Order your own pasta dish from a restaurant (instead of just "trying" someone else's)
- Have a doughnut
- Get a muffin from the bakery with unknown calories
- Order and eat french fries
- Get a burrito from Chipotle, instead of a burrito bowl

Safety Behaviors

As you embark on food exposure with your child, you should be aware of "safety behaviors" your child might engage in to minimize the effect of the exposure, making it less anxiety-inducing. For example, your child might want to weigh their pasta instead of just plating it in order to feel less anxious about eating it. Similarly, they might want to look up the calories in their meal to help them feel more in control, and therefore less anxious. Safety behaviors can interfere with exposure, thus preventing your child from learning to tolerate anxiety during that exposure. For some, removing these safety behaviors will go relatively smoothly, for others it will be much harder. If anxiety levels are so high that your child cannot participate in the exposure, the exposure should be adjusted to something that feels more surmountable.

Here are a few case examples of overcoming safety behaviors.

Case Example: Carmella

Carmella, a seventeen-year-old with resolving bulimia, was about to embark on an ice cream exposure. She chose a local creamery because she knew the calorie count of the ice cream was available online. Knowing the calories made her feel safe, but it also minimized the intensity of the fear. After that experience, the next step was to repeat getting ice cream from an ice cream store where the calories weren't posted. That way she could experience the full feelings of anxiety, to help her learn that nothing bad happened while eating unlabeled ice cream. Carmella seemed up for it, after much discussion, and was able to complete this exposure.

Case Example: Maya

Similarly, Maya only wanted to eat food that was labeled. Throughout the refeeding process, she seemed able to eat everything, until her mother realized that Maya was using the nutrition-fact labels to count calories, to make her feel more safe. Once her parents realized this, they started serving food out of their wrappers. The cereal was moved into clear plastic containers, and more meals were made from scratch or bought from restaurants that did not list nutrition information online. This caused immense anxiety for Maya, whose demeanor reverted back to how she had been early on in treatment. Her parents remembered how they navigated similar situations during Phase 1 of FBT. They knew that Maya's demeanor, with more crying, yelling, sadness, and heightened anxiety, meant they had once again cornered the eating disorder. Just as you didn't let that deter you early on, it shouldn't deter you now. Continuing to reveal the places where your child's eating disorder may still live will only help your child achieve true and lasting recovery.

Case Example: Isa

Isa was working on her fear food, cookies. However, her anxiety kept escalating and she had difficulty breathing just thinking about the exposure. "Cookies are so big," she told the team. Isa had a history of panic attacks, self-harm, and suicidality, and her parents were worried about pushing her too much. They wanted to push her, but felt they needed to take baby steps first. Together with the team, they decided that packaged grocery store cookies, which are smaller than bakery cookies, would be a good first step. Consuming cookies this way allowed Isa to gain confidence with cookies in general—the way it felt in her mouth, the texture, and the taste. After that she would progress to a bakery cookie.

You know your child best, and can decide how and when to push your child. Even children who appear to have high levels of anxiety during this process can be carefully inched along with your commitment to this process.

Additionally, your child's therapist can work with you and your child to formulate a good plan and teach your child coping skills. Coping skills can also be helpful both before and after the food exposure is completed to reduce anxiety. Following is a list of coping tools that can be helpful during times of increased anxiety:

- Have your child take ten deep breaths.
- Engage your child in distracting conversation.
- Watch TV or a movie with your child.
- Have your child take a bath or shower (supervised as needed to prevent treatment-interfering behaviors such as purging or exercise).
- Have your child paint their nails (or yours!).
- Play a board game or work on a puzzle with your child.
- Have your child color, draw, paint, or do an art project.
- Play music for your child.
- Have your child journal about their feelings.
- Have your child knit, sew, or crochet.

To completely eradicate your child's eating disorder, you will become a warrior and fight against your child's avoidance of any foods. You will discover which foods push your child's buttons, and which experiences escalate their anxiety. Your child is unlikely to challenge themselves on their own. To beat the eating disorder, you will need to confidently serve your child the very foods they fear most. You will need to take a loving but firm stance and discontinue catering to the demands of the eating disorder.

As previously discussed, you should approach the table with the expectation that your child *will* eat the food you serve. You do not need to ask your child if they want to try something new. If you ask, "Do you want to try french fries?" most kids struggling with an eating disorder will say no. Instead, say, "Tonight we will have french fries," or you can just serve the fries without encouraging a discussion about it. Your commitment will show your child that you will not accommodate the eating disorder and that you care deeply about their recovery. This will maximize the likelihood that your child will eat what you serve. Of course, they may be angry at you, their anxiety might go up, there might be tears, and they might throw food, but in the end, they won't be scared of the food and will gain the confidence to eat it again.

At the heart of it, successful exposure treatment requires repetition. As you work on repetition, how can you shift the circumstances slightly? If you tried a burger from your grill at home, can you try a burger from a restaurant next time? If you are trying to expose your child to brownies, you might think about how many different ways you can serve a brownie. You might first try baking brownies at home, then buy one from a bakery, and lastly your child may have one at a friend's house. Repeated attempts are important in knocking down the fear and creating new positive experiences. When your child eats the food and "doesn't gain five pounds," they are collecting evidence that can be used to challenge the original irrational thought. Research studying picky eaters shows it can take fifteen to twenty exposures before someone can convert a food from dislike to like.[1] Each exposure is meant to be done many times, in many different forms, and fully experienced (swallowed).

Case Example: Raquel

Raquel, a sixteen-year-old female who had been in a solid state of recovery for around six months, went to her aunt's house for dinner and froze when she learned they were serving lasagna. *Lasagna?* It wasn't until that moment that Raquel realized she was still scared of cheese. She had been eating cold cheese and string cheese regularly, which were no longer scary for her, but at that moment, she realized she was scared of melted cheese that was "gooey and shiny." Somehow, this melted cheese issue had slipped under the radar of her parents and treatment team. Sometimes it takes an experience like eating at your aunt's house or in a restaurant to realize aspects of the eating disorder that are still around. Raquel needed more exposure around eating melted, gooey cheese to help dissolve the fear surrounding it.

When Raquel brought that up in an appointment with her dietitian, she was asked to rank which types of cheese scared her the most. String cheese a 2, quesadillas a 5, and pizza an 8. At this point in recovery, Raquel was more independent and more committed to recovery, so the dietitian asked her to practice making homemade cheese quesadillas. She was able to try that three times in between office visits. She was then asked to rank her anxiety level for quesadillas, and this time her anxiety level was only a 3 (down from a 5). And that was in just a few weeks!

Cognitive Remediation Therapy

The rigidity often seen with eating disorders can also be addressed via techniques that teach mental flexibility and alternate ways of thinking. This is known as cognitive remediation therapy (CRT). According to Camilla Lindvall Dahlgren, PhD, senior researcher at the regional department for eating disorders at Oslo University Hospital in Norway, "In eating disorders, especially in the treatment of anorexia nervosa, CRT is used to help patients become more flexible (less rigid) and to achieve a better balance between bigger picture and detailed thinking." For more than a decade, CRT has been used mainly to treat anorexia nervosa. However, according to Dr. Dahlgren, "Many eating disorders share diagnostic features, and it is therefore likely that CRT could be beneficial in treatment of other eating disorders as well. A number of research trials are currently in progress looking at the effect of CRT in treating both obesity and bulimia nervosa."

With CRT, patients with eating disorders are asked to participate in small behavioral changes to switch up what they do "automatically." For example, perhaps your child can vary their morning routine (eat first and then shower, or vice versa), or perhaps they can sit in a different place at the dinner table. Other examples include brushing your teeth with the less dominant hand, wearing a watch or bracelet on the opposite hand, going makeup free for a day, listening to a different radio station in the car, watching a new TV show, typing your homework in a different font than usual, and last, changing the ringtone of your phone.[2] "Baby steps," Dr. Dahlgren says. "Start with something easy, and take it from there. Change takes time!" Eventually, these activities allow kids to eventually be more flexible, less rigid, and handle subtle changes more easily.

There have been an increasing number of studies looking at the use of CRT with anorexia in adults. Those studies support that CRT decreases rigidity, but randomized clinical trials have not been conducted to date in children and adolescents.[3] In 2010 the original CRT manual, initially used for adults, was reworked for children and adolescents.[4] Though promising, more studies are necessary to evaluate CRT's role in the treatment of eating disorders.

Tackling Areas Where the Eating Disorder Is Still Alive

In order to tackle your child's food vulnerabilities head-on, you will need to have a clear road map of these vulnerabilities. Some will be obvious, and some may be more insidious. In this section, you will find several areas in which kids tend to continue to struggle as they recover. We have included a parent worksheet at the end of this chapter that will help you to summarize key areas in which your child's eating disorder may still be alive.

The best way to understand what you will need to work on with your child is to remember how your child used to eat, before the eating disorder took hold. What were your child's favorite meals? Favorite snacks? Did your child used to love food? Restaurants? Ideally, we want your child to get back to who they were before the onset of the eating disorder. It may seem like an impossible path, but it is possible with dedication and a commitment to taking charge of your child's eating.

For some kids, their nutritional baseline was unbalanced prior to the onset of the eating disorder. Perhaps "before" they had poor nutritional habits and frequently skipped breakfast, grazed all afternoon, or were generally "picky." Or perhaps they relied on fast or frozen food, rather than home-prepared or fresh foods. Their prior habits may have been unbalanced, but their current disordered eating is also unbalanced. In these examples, where the baseline may not have been ideal, it is important to find the middle ground. What aspects can your child borrow from their old way of eating? Typically, if you ask your child, they will say "nothing." But with coaching, they might be able to admit that they liked how they used to be flexible, spontaneous, and that they never worried about food or cared whether their meal timing was off. Most agree that where they have ended up has become too extreme. So how can you push them back into the middle so that they establish healthy eating habits that are not "*too* healthy?"

Letting go of the dietary restrictions

Often with eating disorders, kids will try to plead their case in favor of continuing to adhere to specific dietary restrictions. They may argue about why they should be allowed to remain gluten-free in the absence of a medical diagnosis for celiac disease, dairy-free in the absence of a dairy intolerance, or why they should be allowed to skip desserts during the path to recovery. Your child might make the argument that they "just feel better" without eating gluten or dairy or meat, and this "has nothing to do with the eating disorder." But does it? Here's where your intuition is crucial: does this new development in your child's eating hold them back in some way that they can't overcome? Does your "gluten-free" child eat everything else, such as white rice, brown rice, corn tortilla, quinoa, white potatoes, cereal, etc., easily?

Look out for broad declarations that express extreme rules to be followed "forever." There might be foods your child still tries to avoid. An interest in dietary limitations often emerges for the child at the same time as the eating disorder unfolds. That timing is usually a red flag that the dietary limitation could be intertwined with the eating disorder. And without a clear medical need to avoid something, the treatment team will often recommend that the child include all foods again while their body is healing. This is important since many of the food restrictions and rules prevent the child from getting a sufficient amount of calories, protein, fats, vitamins, and minerals.

Similarly, it could be hard to identify whether your child's newfound vegetarianism is just a strategy to avoid more foods in a socially acceptable way, or whether they are truly passionate about avoiding meat. A fourteen-year-old who has suddenly become passionately committed to vegetarianism may enthusiastically agree to "everything" that is plant-based, in order to be allowed to stay vegetarian. But a person who is hiding behind the vegetarianism to keep an eating disorder alive will remain restrictive, using the vegetarianism to say, "Sorry, I can't eat dinner tonight because I don't eat meat." Or, "I will only eat the spinach at this meal," perhaps because even the beans and rice feel too scary for them. The vegetarian diet could be permitted if, from your point of view, it feels like the development makes sense and represents your child, not their eating disorder. If that's the case, your child should be compliant with following a balanced vegetarian diet. For example, instead of using a barbecue event as a chance to avoid eating, a vegetarian who is recovery-minded might say, "I brought a veggie burger to this barbecue, so I can fill the protein portion of my plate."

Case Example: Zayden

Zayden was always an animal lover. He had three dogs, two cats, fish, and a guinea pig growing up. When his eating disorder was developing, he decided to become a vegan. At this time, he also decided to cut out grains, proteins, and all fats until his diet was mostly vegetables. He quickly became medically unstable and ended up in the hospital.

The hospital couldn't accommodate his vegan diet, because of its limited kitchen, and the treatment team and Zayden's parents decided to compromise on a vegetarian diet instead. This really upset Zayden, but there was no other choice while he was so medically unstable.

Once home, his parents were conflicted about letting him become vegan again. They were worried the diet would be too limited, hold him back from getting enough fuel, and make it hard for him to eat in restaurants, especially during this sensitive time period of recovery. But they knew in their hearts that their son was a long-standing lover of animals and advocate for animal rights. They shared their concerns with Zayden, and ultimately decided they would allow him to follow a vegetarian, not vegan, diet until he recovered. Then, if he was still interested in becoming a vegan, they agreed that he could be free to decide what's best, assuming he maintained his recovery.

Is There Still an Overfocus on Safe, "Clean" Foods?

Xiu vowed that she was recovered but "only wanted" whole-grain breads. "Whole grains are healthier, so why *ever* have white bread? It's a waste of calories," she said.

Other kids may say something similar and hide behind their preferences, "I just don't *like* white bread." But what they are missing is the fact that whole grain options are not always available—so then what? How will your eighteen-year-old go off to college while never eating at a restaurant? Or only eating whole grains? Anything that sounds extreme and unrealistic is usually a red flag that the eating disorder is still breathing right below the surface.

Your child may routinely be sticking to snacks and meals that are "safe," such as a granola bar and a pear, or chicken, kale, and sweet potato. Meals and snacks that are safe are often bland and tasteless, without oils, condiments, or dressings. Those meals may feel "orthorexic" (overly clean and healthy, see chapter 1 for details) or simply just boring! This may sound harsh, but teens with eating disorders often laugh and agree that their meals have become completely repetitive and dull. Often, an eating disorder holds such a firm grip on a child that they have forgotten how to eat. They don't know what they like anymore, they can't tell what looks good, and there is just utter confusion in the kitchen when trying to put together meals. Most parents know in their gut when their child is afraid of something. If your radar is activated, you are probably on to something.

Teens with eating disorders are not healthy, ironically, despite their attempts to eat "clean." As discussed in chapter 1, orthorexic-eating patterns cause kids to become unhealthy both physically and psychologically. The more rules one has around food, the higher the incidence of irritability, depression, anxiety, poor relationships with others, social avoidance, feelings of guilt, and excessive time spent thinking about and/or preparing meals.

Though it might feel unnecessary to fight seemingly minor food restrictions, you should remember that this fight is really about completely obliterating the eating disorder, remnants of which might be lurking in those restrictions.

In an attempt to minimize mealtime fighting, a parent might allow their child to skip something in the meal as long as they eat the rest: "I didn't make her eat the pasta because she ate all her chicken and broccoli." This unfortunately reinforces your child's fear that something is wrong with eating whichever food they avoided that night, and can reinforce the orthorexia in your child. "My child will only eat brown rice, not white rice, and whole wheat pasta, not white pasta, but at least she eats. . . ." Parents are often so relieved to see their child eating that they willingly make these deals with their child, but really, parents are making deals with their child's eating disorder.

The teen might say, "I will drink my milk if I don't have to eat the rice." Or, "I don't like rice, but I will eat quinoa." These negotiations might seem harmless in the moment, especially if the alternative option is calorically equal. But allowing your child to eat these specific food choices perpetuates the child's fears around those foods.

Likewise, many kids may insist they avoid "white foods" and only eat whole grains. However, it is important that your child learn that both types are broken down in the body in a similar way. It is a myth that brown rice is healthier than white rice. It is also a myth that sweet potatoes are healthier than white potatoes. Both types of potatoes contain a variety of nutrients, and both are a healthy addition to the diet. If your child protests, you can present them with these facts:

Myth: Sweet potatoes are healthier than white potatoes.	**Fact:** Potatoes can help a person feel full for a longer period of time, and contain antioxidants (substances that help control oxidative damage in the body) such as carotenoids (vitamin A precursors), ascorbic acid (vitamin C), and tocopherols (vitamin E). Both are high in B vitamins and phytonutrients (nutrients found in plants) such as polyphenols, alpha-lipoic acid, selenium, lycopene, and many more. Fiber is found in the skin and in the insides of both types of potatoes. Sweet potatoes have slightly more fiber per serving, more vitamin A (good for your eyes), manganese (good for wound healing and metabolism), and calcium (good for your bones), but white potatoes have more protein, potassium, and magnesium, and a small amount of iron per serving. Both types of potatoes offer plenty of nutrient density, and both are recommended to be included in the diet.
Myth: Brown rice is healthier than white rice.	**Fact:** While brown rice has more nutrients, such as magnesium, phosphorus, potassium, manganese, selenium, and copper, it also has more calories and carbohydrates than white rice. It also contains phytates, which act as "antinutrients," reducing the ability of the body to utilize and absorb the micronutrients it contains. From a health standpoint, it genuinely is a tie. Neither white rice nor brown rice is superior. Children who consume both white and brown rice get the most nutrients while also remaining flexible.

Is Your Child Eating Enough Variety?

Even as your child progresses, it's important to keep assessing the variety in your child's diet. Take a look back at the seven-day food record that you completed in chapter 6. How often is your child eating the same breakfast? The same lunch? For example, having a yogurt and an apple at snack time might be enough volume for your child, but again, if they are having a yogurt and an apple every day or almost every day, they will remain fearful of other snack foods like pretzels, granola bars, etc. Having cereal and milk every day prevents your child from trying waffles, pancakes, muffins, oatmeal, or eggs. The lack of variety in your child's diet can often pinpoint areas that need improvement.

Eating many foods helps to ensure flexibility, and also helps your body get different nutrients from different foods. For example, chicken is low in iron. If you ate chicken every day, you would be missing out on getting enough iron. Similarly, if you ate an orange every day, you would be missing out on getting the potassium found in bananas.

Below is a sample food record from a teen with an eating disorder. As you can see, they had the same breakfast every morning, and brown

DAILY FOOD RECORD 7/25 → 7/31

MEAL	1	2	3	4	5	6	7
Breakfast	Chia oatmeal 2 eggs 1 cup milk 1 banana ½ avocado	Same	Same	Same	Same	Same	Same
Snack	Blueberries	Blueberries	Blueberries	Grapes	Grapes	Leeches	Strawberries
Lunch	Brown rice Pork Broccoli	Brown rice Chicken Bok choy	Brown rice Pork Green chives	Brown Rice Pork Green Chives	Brown rice chicken mixed veggies	Brown rice fish Kale	Brown rice tofu salmon Bok choy
Snack	Walnuts watermelon	Walnuts watermelon	Cashews	Cashews	Walnuts	Almonds	Walnuts
Dinner	Brown rice Salmon Bok choy	Brown rice tomato fish	Brown rice Bok choy fish	Brown rice Broccoli fish	Potatoes Kale Pork	Brown rice Bok choy fish Tofu	Brown Rice Pork + chicken Broccoli
Snack	None	None	None	None	None	None	None

rice at every lunch and dinner. The format of all of the meals was the same: chicken, pork, or fish, brown rice, and a green vegetable. The morning snack was always a fruit, the afternoon snack was always a type of nut, and they skipped evening snack every night.

Most parents are not gourmet chefs, and often express frustration at running out of meal ideas. They know that the more they can present their child with different options, the better off their child will be in the long run. It can be helpful to plan out what you are serving for dinner in advance, that way you ensure you are varying the proteins, grains/starches, dairy, fruits/vegetables, and fats served.

We often hear parents express the following sentiment, "But my child was never a good eater, they were always picky." Again, the goal is to get back to your child's own baseline, so if they were really picky, they should at least get back to eating what they used to eat. Interestingly though, as this process moves forward, a child with an eating disorder will often start incorporating new foods into their diet, perhaps foods that they never used to like even before the onset of their eating disorder. Developmentally, kids tend to grow out of picky eating as they get older, and frequent exposures help facilitate that and expand their palates.

Last, a fun way to expand what your family eats is to find new recipes. In some cases, using a meal service such as Blue Apron, Hello Fresh, Gobble, Freshly, or Home Chef, can push you out of your comfort zone, in a good way.

Case Example: Nicki

Nicki never liked cheese. During an intensive treatment program, Nicki had to eat what was served to her, or else she would have to drink an Ensure Plus supplement, which made her feel sick. She forced herself a few times to eat the cheese she was served, thinking that eating the cheese was better than drinking the Ensure Plus. It wasn't until months later, that Nicki came in one day and announced, "I ate a quesadilla! I just decided that it was easier to eat cheese for when I go out with my friends, so I worked on it." Her parents were shocked.

Often kids with eating disorders remain fearful when eating out in different restaurants. Challenging your child, especially while you are still so intimately involved in the process can be very beneficial. As you work through different types of eating establishments, don't forget about the key aspects of exposure: repetition and changing the circumstances. Plan to visit all of your old favorite restaurants, and to also include a variety of cuisines such as Mexican, Chinese, Thai, Indian, and Italian. Take your child out for pizza—and master it—by going to different pizza restaurants. Thin-crust pizza is different than deep-dish pizza, and one pizzeria might be different than the next. This is particularly important for older teens, who might be heading off to college, where pizza is a staple, and where take-out is common. It is recommended that you and your child practice eating at buffets, which can often be highly intimidating. This is especially important prior to leaving for college as many college cafeterias are served buffet-style. Another common service type to practice is family-style meals, where large platters are served for everyone to share.

Getting Back to How the Family Eats

When possible, we recommend having the family eat meals together. Research shows having family meals together helps provide kids with support, boundaries, and commitment to learning. Family meals increase your child's social competencies, and help foster a positive identity. Conversely, the fewer family meals had together, the increase in a child's high-risk behaviors, such as substance use, sexual activity, depression/suicide, antisocial behaviors, violence, school problems, binge eating / purging, and excessive weight loss.[5]

It is also important that your child eat the food that is being served at the family meal. If your family is having burgers for dinner, or Chinese food, or going out for ice cream, we would expect your child to join the meal and eat what everyone else is eating. It might be tricky to expect your child to participate in family meal outings prior to being ready (see chapter 13 for eating-on-the-road guidelines). Once in recovery, however, your child should be participating in all of the above and you may need to fight for their attendance at these meals or events. Imagine if your child was "recovered" and refusing to go out with the whole family for ice cream. How would that feel to you? It might make you think twice about how solid their recovery is.

Case Example: Sonali

Sonali's family eats Indian food every night for dinner. They were upset because after the onset of her eating disorder, she refused to eat her mom's homemade Indian cooking, opting instead for something she made herself. Sonali didn't like how much oil her mother used when making the food and thought it was too "fattening." Her treatment team suggested to Sonali that her avoidance of Indian food seemed driven by her fears. She was scared about "what the Indian food would do to her body."

After a long discussion about why fats were important for her body, and the importance of tackling all foods that scare her, Sonali reluctantly agreed to eat what her family was eating. Through a discussion between the dietitian, parents, and Sonali, a decision was reached that as long as she was eating some Indian food with the family each week, she didn't have to eat it seven out of seven days. After all, Sonali was seventeen and was going off to college soon, where she wouldn't be able to have Indian food every night anyway. Her parents agreed it made more sense to allow Sonali to practice eating all kinds of foods at night, as long as she was working on increasing exposure (and eventually acceptance) of Indian cooking.

In some circumstances, returning to "the family's baseline" might not be possible or recommended. An obvious example of this would be for a family where there is no cohesive meal structure. Many families don't eat together out of schedule necessity—one person eats at 6:00 p.m. before dance practice, another eats at 8:00 p.m. after soccer, Mom eats somewhere in between, and Dad eats at work. Or, if family members have medical concerns such as diabetes or heart disease, the adolescent without those diagnoses should not mimic their parents' diet. A parent may have an eating disorder, in which case, eating how their parent eats might be exactly what the teen is trying to move away from. In divorced households, one parent might eat one way and another might eat in another way. The goal, when "getting back to how the family eats" is not ideal, is to help the teen sculpt their own food identity, that feels balanced, healthy (but not *too* healthy), and that supports their medical and nutritional goals.

In very health-conscious families, there may be a list of foods the family as a whole chooses to avoid. The more health conscious a family is, the harder it is to meet the goals of nutritional rehabilitation for a child with an eating disorder. Michele Vivas, MS, RD, a well-known eating disorder specialist says, "The rules for a starving body, are different than for a fed body." An undernourished body that is exhibiting signs of malnutrition such as low heart rate, amenorrhea, or cold hands, needs a high-caloric, high-fat diet, and quickly. Families in health-conscious or sugar-free households can accomplish the goals of refeeding by getting creative with lots of nuts and avocados. Unfortunately, day after day, this can quickly become repetitive and limited. While families can customize meals and purchase specialty ingredients, it becomes less realistic for teenagers to do so on their own as they begin to navigate the world. College cafeterias might not be able to cater to such a specific diet. Or as a child becomes more self-sufficient, it might be too expensive for them to adhere to those same guidelines once on their own. One of the best gifts a parent can give their child as it relates to food is the ability to be flexible.

Meal Ideas to Inspire Variety

Recovery offers a period of growth as it relates to one's relationship with food. A child doing the work of exposure, variety, and reintroduction of food groups may end up being willing to try all kinds of foods, sometimes even food their family doesn't eat. The path to rebuilding one's relationship with food might involve food discoveries that lead them to stray out of the family boundaries a little. A child recovering from an eating disorder may discover that they *want* to eat sugar (even if their family doesn't) or they *want* to eat meat (even if their family doesn't), in the spirit of openness, flexibility, and establishing a solid recovery.

Parent Worksheet: Letting Go of Food Fears

1. How does your child's current diet compare to their diet *before* the onset of the eating disorder? What were your child's favorite meals when they were younger?

2. How varied is your child's diet in the following categories? Brainstorm new foods that you can add to your child's meals.

_____

Grains/starches

_____

Proteins

_____

Fruits

_____

Vegetables

_____

Fats

_____

Dairy

_____

Fluids

_____

Snacks

3. What foods are considered "safe" to your child?

4. What are your child's "fear foods?" Can you rank these fear foods in a hierarchy from least to most scary? Using a chart like the one below can be helpful. To do this, rate each food on a scale of 1–10 (1 = not scary and 10 = terrifying!). Remember, it can take fifteen to twenty times of trying the same food over and over before your child begins to feel more comfortable. You can track how many times you try each food by marking the boxes under "number of tries." You/your child can also track anxiety levels before and after each exposure using the log below.

DATE	FEAR FOOD	ANXIETY RATING *BEFORE* EXPOSURE	ANXIETY RATING *AFTER* EXPOSURE
For Example: 8/20/2018	Croissant	8	6

5. Eating at Restaurants

Put a check box if your child has eaten in the following types of restaurants, and keep track of how many times you have tried it.

FOOD	NUMBER OF TRIES											
CHINESE RESTAURANT 1												
CHINESE RESTAURANT 2												
MEXICAN FOOD 1												
MEXICAN FOOD 2												
PIZZA PLACE 1												
PIZZA PLACE 2												
BURGER FROM RESTAURANT												
BURGER FROM HOME												
SANDWICH SHOP 1												
SANDWICH SHOP 2												
BUFFET LINE 1												
BUFFET LINE 2												

CHAPTER 15

Returning to Normal

Phase 3 of FBT

AS YOU'RE DRIVING to what feels like your child's three hundredth nutrition appointment, you find yourself thinking, "Do we even need to keep going to these appointments? My child eats everything I put on their plate and has been successful with eating independently for a while! I can't remember the last time they had a meltdown about food." If this resonates with you, welcome to Phase 3 of FBT! This is great news and a testament to you and your child's hard work throughout this process. But this is not the time to step on the brakes. Rather, it's the perfect time to shake things up and lead your child through the next (and hopefully last) phase of treatment.

Up until this point, your child has likely been following the Plate-by-Plate approach to eating: three meals and two or three snacks per day, at very specific times. They have been finishing 100 percent of their plate with your complete supervision (Phase 1 of FBT). Your child might have progressed to plating some of their own meals and snacks, with your supervision, once they became weight restored (Phase 2 of FBT). And now, you have landed in Phase 3.

By the time you reach this phase of treatment, you might be exhausted. It most likely hasn't been easy. You and your child probably struggled in the beginning—and the middle—and you may still struggle from time to time even today. By now however, the meltdowns are less frequent, and you and your child have *got this*. That beast of an eating disorder that reared its ugly head at every meal in the beginning is now quiet, managed, and hardly around. By now your child even has a few tools to battle the eating disorder on their own when it tries to creep back in. After all of the fighting around food and all of the stress, there is finally less to worry about. Your child is now weight-restored, eating regular meals and snacks, and beginning to rediscover the joy of eating.

You might be thinking, "Why rock the boat now? This is the first time in months or even years that the dinner table has returned to its mostly calm state." There is still some important work left to do, and it is a pivotal and very necessary part of eating disorder treatment. This next phase, the transition to "normal eating," helps your child:

- Regain a **sense of normalcy around eating**
- Become an **independent eater** again
- Learn to **trust their body** to guide their eating choices, rather than relying on you and the treatment team to tell them what, when, and how to eat
- Finally **reclaim food freedom** and become **a fearless eater**

What Is Normal Eating?

Our goal during this process is to teach your child how to eat normally again. This includes learning to respond to their hunger cues so they can eat when they are hungry and stop when they are full. Internationally recognized expert on feeding and eating Ellyn Satter, MS, RD, describes the following characteristics of "normal eating"[1]:

- Going to the table hungry and eating until you are satisfied
- Being able to choose food you like, eat it, and truly get enough of it; not stopping because you think you should
- Being able to give some thought to your food selection so you get nutritious food, but not being so wary and restrictive that you miss out on enjoyable food
- Giving yourself permission to eat sometimes because you are happy, sad, or bored, or just because it feels good

- Eating mostly three meals a day, or four or five, or choosing to munch along the way
- Leaving some cookies on the plate because you know you can have some again tomorrow, or eating more now because they taste so wonderful
- Overeating at times, feeling stuffed and uncomfortable
- Undereating at times and wishing you had more
- Trusting your body to make up for your mistakes in eating
- Letting eating take up some of your time and attention, but keeping its place as only one important area of your life

In short, normal eating is flexible. It varies in response to your hunger, your schedule, your proximity to food, and your feelings.

It can take a long time for kids who have battled eating disorders to reach that level of normalcy around eating. You might first see glimmers of it as your child begins to graze or pick at food between meals, ask for their old favorites again, show signs of enjoying food, and eat spontaneously. These are signs that your child is shifting away from rigidity and obsessiveness and moving toward fearless eating. We wait a long time for those behaviors to emerge, and they are usually a great indicator that your child is heading in the right direction.

How to Know When Your Child Is Ready

Before normal eating behaviors can resume, your child must be out of medical danger. Maintaining medical stability, as indicated by weight, vital signs, and blood work, means that your child's mental and physical state are in a safe and healthy place. When your child is at a healthy weight, their heart and brain are sufficiently nourished. Their metabolism has probably also normalized, allowing them to correctly understand their hunger and satiety cues. By this point, your child's anxiety around food is generally greatly reduced, despite your child being at a higher weight. If your child's weight continues to fluctuate, or to remain below the projected goal weight provided by the treatment team, then your child is likely not ready to begin this next phase.

Along the same lines, once medically stable and weight-restored, female teens usually start to see their periods resume. That said, many factors can affect the menstrual cycle, such as stress, diet, hormonal imbalances, and energy expenditure. Working with a medical provider and a dietitian is important to understanding why your child's menstrual period is either irregular or absent. Resumption of menses can take up to six months after achieving weight restoration.[2]

If your child is not getting regular periods but meets the other criteria listed in this chapter, then we suggest a careful discussion with the treatment team to determine if your child is ready for this next phase. For some, skipped periods will be a lingering sign that their energy balance is not yet stable. Perhaps your child is exercising too much and not eating enough, or not consuming enough dietary fats. In those cases, you might want to wait to make changes to meals. For others, their weight and mindset may be in a great place, but their menstrual cycles and hormone levels will need time to return. Your child's physician can do lab work to check current estradiol levels, which indicate how close they are to getting their period back. If mentally your child appears to be in a good place, and if they are exhibiting some of the signs of normal eating listed below, it is possible to begin the transition to normal eating despite lack of menses. For boys, you can test their medical vital signs, testosterone levels, and psychological mindset to determine whether they are ready.

Gaining Confidence

In addition to medical stability, another important factor in order for your child to transition to normal eating is gauging the degree to which the eating disorder still has a hold over your child, if at all. Are you confident that your child can finish meals when you are not present? Some parents will have an immediate reaction to that question. "No way." Or "definitely." Others may be unsure. If you're not sure of the answer, now is the time to "test" the eating disorder's grip by allowing more and more freedom. When done in tandem with frequent medical check-ins (which should continue even throughout this last phase), you can get a sense of whether your child's increased freedom will be a threat to their continued health.

When you give them more freedom at meals, are they able to maintain their weight? Does the menstrual cycle remain regular? Before beginning the return to normal eating, you should know whether your child will successfully complete a meal or snack when no one is watching. If your child engages in eating-disorder behaviors such as hiding food or leaving food behind, then it is clear that the eating disorder is still alive. In this case your child will need to continue with the supervised meals and snacks for a while longer.

What to Do If the Eating Disorder Still Has a Firm Grip on Your Child

1. **Is your child really at the right weight?** Have your team reassess your child's growth curve. Often, treatment continues for a long time, and as a child ages and grows, expectations for weight gain increase. The treatment goals for weight provided by your team early on might need to be adjusted.

2. **Can you work on more food exposure?** Those who are struggling might need to work on increasing exposure to fear foods. Refer to chapter 14 for details. A renewed focus on increasing variety will help your child become more flexible with food.

3. **Set small, achievable goals** such as "eating one meal at a restaurant" or "trying one new food" this weekend.

4. **Work on increasing your child's independence around food.** Try allowing your child to choose an evening snack at night or to plate a meal on their own, with your official sign-off.

5. **Practice choosing "yummy" foods.** Your child may still be bound by calories. Take Leah, for example. Leah would look up the calories of all meals, choosing whichever had the least. Leah was asked by her treatment team to do the opposite: to go to a restaurant, sit with the menu, and just order what sounded "yummy." Practicing these skills paves the way for normal eating.

Greater Comfort Around Food

Once your child is physically in a healthy place, they may begin to request certain foods. Suddenly, the child who swore they would never eat your shepherd's pie asks for it one day. They may also ask for "those cookies that Aunt Bonnie makes" or "your famous mac and cheese." At this point, you might be trying hard not to let your mouth hang open in disbelief. During this stage, kids may finally begin to feel comfortable in a restaurant. Ordering from a menu becomes easier. This is the reward that comes from all of your hard work in Phases 1 and 2.

By this time, your child has likely become so used to "exposure, exposure, exposure" that eventually all foods become fair game. They can finally taste the flavors in food without feeling stressed and can finally explore different food choices without the fear that those foods are going to make them fat. Somewhere along the way to eating more, gaining weight, and checking in with medical providers, it happened: your child actually started to like food again!

Your child may have also started eating spontaneously again. For example, they may try a bite of your entrée at a restaurant one night, something they never would have done before because that would have been "extra." Or they may have a brownie at school because someone brought them in for a birthday celebration, despite the fact that they already had their morning snack. They may start to graze, such as grabbing a handful of pretzels before dinner or taking some nuts that were in a bowl on the counter after lunch. These new behaviors are often shocking to parents and are a great signal that their child is moving forward. Parents may secretly wonder, is this okay? The answer is an unqualified yes. This is part of the process of returning to normal eating.

Flexibility around food generally increases during this time. Flexibility means your child is eating different foods each day—different breakfasts, lunches, dinners, and snacks—and there may be less of a specific pattern into which your child's eating falls. Sudden meal changes that may result from running out of something or being unable to go to the store don't rattle your child as they did before. For example, if you send your child with ham instead of turkey in their sandwich, they are fine with that substitution. If your child goes to a friend's house for dinner, there will be no concern about what food is being served that night. If the food has some oil on it, your child doesn't complain anymore.

Your child may still have body-image concerns, but we find that at this point, those concerns no longer drive your child's actions around food. While your child may express dissatisfaction with their body, generally they are now able to separate how they feel about their body from their food intake.

Case Example: Dani

Dani is a fifteen-year-old girl whose weight dropped from 106 down to 90 pounds. Her initial goal weight was set at 105–110 pounds, but when she reached that goal weight, it turned out she had grown 1.5 inches. The goal weight was increased to 115–120 pounds to account for that growth. With a lot of hard work, she finally reached her new goal weight range, and after a long struggle, she was finally in a much improved mental space.

One day, there was a new medical assistant working with her doctor. The new medical assistant left Dani's weight that day on the counter for her to see. It was an innocent mistake, but one that could have been devastating for Dani in previous phases of treatment—one that in the past would have likely led to relapse. Dani shared with the team that knowing she had "gained *that much* weight" made her feel uncomfortable but she was still committed to recovery and wasn't going to "take it out on her food."

Testing the waters

To decide if your child is ready for this next step, some (if not all) of these behaviors should be present, along with medical stabilization. Spontaneous eating, even if it happens only once or twice, demonstrates that your child is moving in the right direction. Asking for a second helping or adding something to their meal means that they are no longer adhering to rigid food rules. Making food requests demonstrates an interest in food again. These behaviors will happen naturally, *when the child is ready*. Once these positive eating behaviors occur, your child can safely work toward a more flexible and normal style of eating.

For some kids, the decision to shift toward normal eating is an obvious next step. Alex is a fourteen-year-old girl who, after a long battle with anorexia, is medically stable, in a healthy goal-weight range, and getting regular periods; she has just begun eating spontaneously in between meals. Her mother marveled, "She's even taking a little extra!" Alex's parents now finally feel confident that if they leave her alone for a meal, she will be able to eat all of it. She seems ready for this next step. However, in other cases, the treatment team may need to "test out" this next phase and push the child along.

Small tests, whether it's going to a new restaurant, traveling, or allowing a sleepover, are all experiences that provide you with information about your child's recovery. Can your child be successful under those circumstances? Did you learn something new about your child's lingering food and weight fears from the experiment? Though it was exhausting to get here, your child is now weight restored, which helps to give them a "buffer." As they progress, they are also becoming more resilient and are likely to be more capable of getting back on track should they get derailed. As parents, you have become savvy and experienced at managing your child's eating-disorder recovery. Unlike at the beginning of treatment, you can now instantly recognize the warning signs that something is off and you have the tools to steer your child back to the right path.

Parents are often apprehensive to experiment with greater food autonomy and normalcy because their child has improved so much, and they don't want to disrupt the balance that they have worked so hard to achieve. However, if your child is not encouraged to take these last few steps on their own, they may not ever fully recover. In experimenting with food autonomy during this phase, you'll gain insight into your child's resiliency, an important skill for eating-disorder recovery and normal eating.

Is Your Child Ready for "Normal Eating"?

Your child is ready to take this next step when they:
- Consistently maintain medical stability, staying within a healthy weight range (REQUIRED)
- Can eat and complete at least one unsupervised meal per day (REQUIRED)
- Are getting regular periods
- Enjoy food again
- Make requests for foods they used to love
- Can eat spontaneously (i.e., asking for a few pieces of chocolate after dinner)
- Are more flexible with food, eating what is served without complaint
- Can eat out at a restaurant without heightened anxiety or stress

Identifying and Responding to Hunger Cues

If your child is ready to progress to normal eating, they must learn to understand their hunger and satiety cues. Think about a holiday meal or the last time you ate at a restaurant. More than likely, you left the table feeling full or perhaps outright uncomfortable. This is not uncommon, and the feeling probably passed after about an hour or so. To you, that may not have been a very big deal; you may not have even thought twice about it. But to a child with an eating disorder, that feeling can be devastating. Teaching a child to be a more intuitive eater starts with a discussion about hunger and fullness.

In the earlier stages of treatment, it is very common for a child with an eating disorder to say they just don't feel any hunger or fullness cues: "I only feel full; I never feel hungry." This is partly due to the physiological changes that occur during the refeeding process, plus the high volume of food required for weight gain. Anxiety around food can also inhibit a person's hunger levels. Being at a stable weight and on a regular schedule of meals allows your child to get in touch with their body again. However, it may still be possible that your child does not recognize these cues.

Your child may be used to feeling extreme hunger (from periods of food restriction) and has come to perceive that as "normal" hunger. Alternatively, your child may be very sensitive to hunger and perceive a small pang of hunger as a sign they aren't eating enough. We expect that prior to meals and snacks kids will feel hungry; it is a signal that it's nearing time to eat. Fluctuating levels of hunger are completely normal and should occur regularly throughout the day. "Feeling full" is normal and usually passes thirty to sixty minutes after a meal.

To master this part, your child can begin to track their hunger levels throughout the day. This is best done with the help of a registered dietitian who will guide your child through this process. Your child can rate their hunger levels on a scale of 1 to 10, with 1 being not hungry at all and 10 being extremely hungry. Initially, your child may struggle to decipher what their body is feeling. But with practice, your child will begin to understand the different intensity levels of their hunger. They will compare how they felt at breakfast to how they felt at lunch, and again at dinner. And slowly, your child will be reacquainted with their appetite.

Before a meal or snack, your child's hunger level should be around levels 5 to 7. Ideally, your child will be hungry, but not starving. If your child reaches a 10 on the hunger scale before their meal, that is a clear sign that they didn't eat enough at the last meal. Following a regular schedule, where your child continues to eat every three to four hours, will help stimulate their appetite while preventing hunger levels from becoming too extreme.

Some kids go through this process and still struggle to feel hunger. They may say they are "never hungry" or they "don't remember what hunger feels like because they're always eating." In this situation, the dietitian may ask a child to instead explore fullness levels instead. They may be asked to rate their fullness on a scale of 1 to 10, with 1 being not full, 5 being satisfied, and 10 being extremely full or uncomfortable. After eating a typical meal, their fullness level should hover around 5. There may be times, though, when their meal was slightly too small and they aren't full (level 1). Or they went to a new restaurant with larger plates than what you use at home and feel "stuffed" afterward (level 10). Asking your child this will help them pay attention to normal body cues and adjust food intake appropriately, even if they say they don't recognize hunger yet.

This phase of treatment is more of an art than a science. It takes time, practice, and a lot of patience from all involved. It will be bumpy, scary, and awkward sometimes, but in time, it will lead your child to be a truly normal eater.

Meal Guidelines for Normal Eating

A child transitioning to normal eating will need rough guidelines to follow so that the eating disorder doesn't lead them astray during this phase.

Your child should still stick to a schedule of "three meals and two or three snacks" where all food groups are present. Meals and snacks should be spaced no more than three hours apart. This is your child's road map and will help them reconnect with their intuitive hunger and fullness cues. It also won't change—in fact, we recommend this meal structure for most people, whether you are recovering from an eating disorder or not. Eating regularly keeps blood sugar levels stable throughout the day, keeps hunger in the desired range (preventing over- and undereating), and improves energy and concentration.

The next step is allowing some flexibility with how much your child "has to" finish at mealtime. Before, your child was expected to eat 100 percent of food on the plate. Now, your child should check in with their body before, during, and after the meal, to decide how much they need to eat. Your child will need to consider their level of hunger or fullness after they have completed about 75 percent of their plate (less than that may signal food restriction). Are they full? Still hungry? Do they want more? How does their stomach feel? If your child decides they are genuinely full, they can stop eating at this point. This is especially helpful for restaurant meals, which might be more calorically dense, so completing 100 percent of a meal is less intuitive. Interestingly, most of the time, kids continue to eat 100 percent of their plates even once granted this new freedom because they are truly hungry and because the food *tastes* good. This shift may take you by surprise because it is so different than what you have become accustomed to during this process. However, allowing your child to leave behind some food or to have second helpings if they wish strengthens their own intuition around food.

Those who eat 75 percent at one meal and stop there should be aware that they may be hungrier at the next meal. They might therefore eat 125 percent at the next meal, asking for seconds. This can be a very challenging process and will take a lot of practice and encouragement. Your child will likely second-guess themselves: "Did I eat too much?" or "Do I still need more?" There is much more room for interpretation in this phase than before, when meals needed to be completed 100 percent. In time, however, your child will make their way toward eating intuitively and normally.

Be an observer. This is the first time in treatment that your child gets to decide how much they need, which can be scary for you both. Try not to comment on the amount your child consumes, and allow them to test out this new way of eating. If your child spontaneously asks for a food item (e.g., a cookie or a piece of fruit) before the next scheduled meal or snack time, allow them to have it.

Expect your child to still eat a minimum of 75 percent at the next meal or snack. If they are too full because they had that extra food item, let them know they still need to eat 75 percent (that's the rule at this point). Remind yourself that it's okay for your child to be more full and that they will learn to listen to their body more closely the next time. This is how a child learns to self-regulate hunger and fullness. It is also how parents and the treatment team prevent the eating disorder from creeping back into mealtime.

Don't expect perfection. This phase of treatment is not only about what your child is learning to do differently but also about what *you* are learning to do differently. It is the beginning of a new period of trial and error with food. Your child may get it "right" some of the time, and they may get it "wrong" some of the time. That's okay. The main goal is to allow them to explore hunger and fullness cues again and to practice as they learn how to eat *normally*.

As this process continues, allow your child to make reasonable food requests based on foods they used to love and may have restricted in earlier phases of treatment. For example, if your child used to love Baskin-Robbins ice cream, go get a scoop or two. If they have been hesitant to try pepperoni pizza, order delivery! The key here is to normalize everything and to support your child in becoming a more adventurous eater again. As you hear appropriate and *normal* food comments (e.g., "Yum! That cookie was sooo good," or "Hey, can you please make that macaroni casserole again?"), you can entertain additional food requests. Perhaps your child wants carrots and hummus for a snack. In the past, asking for carrots would have seemed like a request from your child's eating disorder and not their true preference. But if you have heard your child routinely ask for other, scarier foods, it is more likely your child *truly likes* carrots with hummus. If that is the case, and your gut tells you the request is coming from a genuine place (and is not an eating-disorder request), then go ahead and allow it. Your child will quickly become empowered to communicate with you about foods they like.

A Parent's Guide to the Do's and Don'ts of Normal Eating

DO...	DON'T...
Stick to a schedule of three meals and two or three snacks per day	Worry about your child continuing to gain weight; this is normal and it will stabilize
Continue to follow the Plate-by-Plate approach	Let fear of relapse prevent you from experimenting with food autonomy in this phase
Let your child make reasonable food requests	Limit your child's access to sweets; allow the exposure to normalize eating
Make sure your child eats at least 75 percent of meals and snacks	Stop supervising meals and snacks unless recommended to do so by the team
Allow your child to have second helpings and eat less than 100 percent if they want to	Allow your child to plan and shop for meals and snacks unless recommended by the team
Allow spontaneous eating between meals and snacks as long as it doesn't interfere with completing the next meal or snack	Talk about "good" foods versus "bad" foods; all foods are good foods in the right balance

Making the Transition

Let's walk through how you and your child's treatment team may begin to approach this topic of transitioning to "normal" eating so you are familiar with it when the time comes. The dialogue between your child and the team should go something like this:

Clinician: "I am hearing from you and your parents that you are completing one hundred percent of your meals and snacks, you are eating flexibly, and sometimes even spontaneously. You are getting regular periods and your vital signs are rock-solid stable. This is a sign that you are getting the right amount of food. This is also a sign that you are ready to have some independence with food."

Child: "Really?"

Clinician: "Yep! We will take baby steps with the end goal being that you can choose how much to eat based on your body's hunger and fullness signals."

Child: "Umm, I don't really know what hunger feels like anymore, and I'm scared I won't be able to trust my body."

Clinician: "That's okay and normal at this stage. We [your team and parents] have been doing the decision making for you because we didn't trust your eating disorder and your hunger and satiety cues were suppressed due to malnutrition. Now that you have more control over your eating disorder, we want to teach you how to listen to your body again so that you can eat intuitively and normally."

Child: "What is *normal* eating anyway?"

Clinician: "While there is a wide variety of what is considered *normal*—generally speaking it is getting enough food to truly satisfy hunger. It is not restrictive, nor impulsive. Some thought goes into eating but it is not an all-consuming process. It can be missing meals occasionally because you didn't plan properly and making up for a missed meal by eating more at the next. It can be eating more than you need sometimes because the food tastes so good, or because you are bored, emotional, or tired, and it is learning from those experiences and trusting your body to fill in the gaps."[3]

Child: "That sounds normal, but I'm so afraid of it for some reason."

Clinician: "It's okay to be scared and nervous about this change; it's a big change and it's a necessary step in your recovery."

Child: "Okay, I guess I can give it a try."

Clinician: "Great. Here's how we'll begin. I want you to continue eating three meals and two or three snacks per day. The difference is that now you are allowed to leave some food on your plate if you feel satisfied at that point. You're also allowed to ask for more food if you feel unsatisfied after finishing your plate. The goal is for you to eat at least seventy-five percent of your plate, and you can use your hunger and fullness levels to decide how much more to eat beyond that. There is no right answer at any particular meal, only trial and error. I will ask your parents and you to report back to me about how the meals are going. This will take time, and it may be very uncomfortable at first; however, the more you practice the more comfortable and natural this will become."

Child: "Can I skip any meals if I am not hungry?"

Clinician: "No. Your body is still fragile, and skipping meals can be a very slippery road to relapse. Plus, it is recommended for all people, with or without an eating disorder, to eat meals every three to four hours throughout the day. This way the body gets the right amount of food and it prevents over- and undereating. For now, stick to the same eating schedule and only change the amount you complete based on your hunger and fullness levels. The amount you eat will vary from one meal to the next and one day to the next. That is normal as well."

Child: "Okay, I will try this out."

Clinician: "Great, see you next week!"

Trouble Signs

As you and your child embark on this new leg of the journey, there are some red flags to watch out for:

- Your child consistently eats only the bare minimum (75 percent) at meals and snacks. That is a sign they are not eating based on their intuition, and instead are likely eating based on food rules the eating disorder has created.
- Your child's food variety is narrowing, and they consistently choose "safe" foods reminiscent of earlier stages of treatment.
- You catch your child hiding food or trying to "get out of" eating something.
- At medical check-ins, you discover your child is consistently losing weight.
- Increased frequency of arguments or negotiations at mealtime. This may be a sign that the eating disorder is still too strong for this phase of treatment.

These red flags do not necessarily mean that your child cannot move forward with this more normal way of eating. They might, however, mean that your child needs to practice in a more limited way—for example, only at dinnertime under your direct guidance. Sometimes a more gradual approach is necessary for this transition to be successful and effective. Either way, good communication with the treatment team about what you observe during this third phase of treatment is key. And while the end goal is to help your child reestablish autonomy with food, the path is usually not linear. Your child might struggle during this phase; they may need to return to a more structured meal plan with direct supervision from you before being truly ready to practice eating in this way. However, it is important to continue guiding your child in this direction toward "normal eating."

Closing Thoughts

If you have made it to this point, congratulations! You and your child have done a tremendous amount of work. You have fought a long and arduous battle with a deadly beast of a disease, and you have saved your child from the grip of an eating disorder. Getting your child to eat "normally" again is a huge accomplishment and you should feel relieved to have your child *back*! And while you may be finished with this book, remember that the Plate-by-Plate model will always be a tool you and your child can rely on to stay on track with food.

Recovery takes several months, if not years, to solidify. Don't be surprised if your child's recovery includes some ups and downs. There may be tears the first time your child tries on a bathing suit, or when they have to throw away their favorite old jeans. The difference now is that your child has become more resilient in the face of these obstacles, and more committed to their recovery. And they know firsthand the dangers associated with taking their emotions out on their food or their body. At some point, your child will be truly free to eat however they wish. Yet they will always need to be thoughtful about large changes in their diet.

As a parent, you will be there to help when the road gets bumpy. Relapse can happen. What's important is that you and your child now have the skills to stay ahead of the eating disorder, to notice where it may hide, to be curious about changes in eating and exercise behaviors, and to "go back to what worked" at any point should recovery shift to relapse. Hopefully, your child will maintain a fully recovered life, made possible by all of the effort put toward treatment, and this eating disorder will keep its place as only one scary chapter of your child's otherwise healthy and happy life.

To all of the parents out there, we salute you! Your child could not beat this illness without you.

NOTES

Introduction

1. E. G. Nicdao, S. Hong, and D. T. Takeuchi, "Prevalence and Correlates of
    Eating Disorders Among Asian Americans: Results from the National
    Latino and Asian American Study," *International Journal of Eating
    Disorders* 40, supplement (November 2007): S22–26.

    J. Y. Taylor, C. H. Caldwell, R. E. Baser, et al., "Prevalence of Eating
    Disorders Among Blacks in the National Survey of American Life,"
    International Journal of Eating Disorders 40, supplement (November
    2007): S10–14.

    K. T. Eddy, M. Hennessey, and H. Thompson-Brenner, "Eating Pathology
    in East African Women: The Role of Media Exposure and Globalization,"
    Journal of Nervous and Mental Disease 195, no. 3 (March 2007): 196–202.

    L. Marques, M. Alegria, A. E. Becker, et al., "Comparative Prevalence,
    Correlates of Impairment, and Service Utilization for Eating Disorders
    Across US Ethnic Groups: Implications for Reducing Ethnic Disparities in
    Health Care Access for Eating Disorders," *International Journal of Eating
    Disorders* 44, no. 5 (July 2011): 412–20.

    M. Alegria, M. Woo, Z. Cao, et al., "Prevalence and Correlates of Eating
    Disorders in Latinos in the United States," *International Journal of Eating
    Disorders* 40, supplement (November 2007): S15–21.

    Matthew B. Feldman and Ilan H. Meyer, "Eating Disorders in Diverse
    Lesbian, Gay, and Bisexual Populations," *International Journal of Eating
    Disorders* 40, no. 3 (April 2007): 218–26, doi:10.1002/eat.20360.

    N. Chisuwa and J. A. O'Dea, "Body Image and Eating Disorders Amongst
    Japanese Adolescents: A Review of the Literature," *Appetite* 54, no. 1
    (February 2010): 5–15.

    "Position Paper of the Society for Adolescent Health and Medicine:
    Medical Management of Restrictive Eating Disorders in Adolescents and
    Young Adults," *Journal of Adolescent Health* 56, no. 1 (January 2015):
    121–25, doi:10.1016/j.jadohealth.2014.10.259.

P. S. Chandra, S. Abbas, R. Palmer, "Are Eating Disorders a Significant Clinical Issue in Urban India? A Survey Among Psychiatrists in Bangalore," *International Journal of Eating Disorders* 45, no. 3 (April 2012): 443–46.

S. Lee, K. L. Ng, K. Kwok, et al., "The Changing Profile of Eating Disorders at a Tertiary Psychiatric Clinic in Hong Kong (1987–2007)," *International Journal of Eating Disorders* 43, no. 4 (May 2010): 307–14.

T. Jackson and H. Chen, "Sociocultural Experiences of Bulimic and Non-bulimic Adolescents in a School-Based Chinese Sample," *Journal of Abnormal Child Psychology* 38, no. 1 (January 2010): 69–76.

2. S. F. Forman, L. F. Grodin, D. A. Graham, et al., "An Eleven Site National Quality Improvement Evaluation of Adolescent Medicine-Based Eating Disorder Programs: Predictors of Weight Outcomes at One Year and Risk Adjustment Analyses," *Journal of Adolescent Health* 49, no. 6 (December 2011): 594–600.

Chapter 1: Understanding Eating Disorders and the Obsession with Food

1. American Psychiatric Association, *Diagnostic and Statistical Manual of Mental Disorders*, 5th ed. (Washington, DC: American Psychiatric Association, 2013).

2. "Binge Eating Disorder," National Eating Disorders Association, nationaleatingdisorders.org/binge-eating-disorder.

3. Newsweek Staff, "The Pressure to Lose," *Newsweek*, May 1, 1994, newsweek .com/pressure-lose-188802.

4. D. Neumark-Sztainer and PJ Hannan. "Weight-Related Behaviors Among Adolescent Girls and Boys: A National Survey," Archives of Pediatric and Adolescent Medicine, 154, no. 6 (June 2001): 569–77.

    K. Boutelle, D. Neumark-Sztainer, M. Story, and M. Resnick, "Weight Control Behaviors Among Obese, Overweight, and Nonoverweight Adolescents," *Journal of Pediatric Psychology* 27, no. 6 (September 2002): 531–40.

5. E. Wertheim, S. Paxton, and S. Blaney, "Body Image in Girls," in L. Smolak and J. K. Thompson, eds., *Body Image, Eating Disorders, and Obesity in Youth: Assessment, Prevention, and Treatment*, 2nd ed. (Washington, DC: American Psychological Association, 2009), 47–76.

6. D. Neumark-Sztainer, *"I'm, Like, SO Fat!": Helping Your Teen Make Healthy Choices about Eating and Exercise in a Weight-Obsessed World* (New York: Guilford, 2005).

7. A. Keys, J. Brožek, A. Henschel, O. Mickelsen, and H. L. Taylor, *The Biology of Human Starvation*, 2 volumes (St. Paul: University of Minnesota Press, 1950).

8. D. Le Grange, E. C. Accurso, J. Lock, S. Agras, S. W. Bryson, "Early Weight Gain Predicts Outcome in Two Treatments for Adolescent Anorexia Nervosa," *International Journal of Eating Disorders* 47, no. 2 (March 2014): 124–29, doi: 10.1002/eat.22221. Epub November 4, 2013.

9. Almeida, Liliana, "Reduce Body Checking With Two Easy Steps," Very Well Mind, last modified January 14, 2018, verywell.com/reduce-body-checking-with-two-easy-steps-1138366?utm_source=emailshare&utm_medium=social&utm_campaign=shareurlbuttons.

10. Bonnie A. Spear, Sarah E. Barlow, Chris Ervin, David S. Ludwig, Brian E. Saelens, Karen E. Schetzina, and Elsie M. Taveras, "Recommendations for Treatment of Child and Adolescent Overweight and Obesity, Pediatrics Supplement," *Pediatrics* 120, supplement 4 (December 2007): 164–92, doi:10.1542/peds.2007-2329F.

11. C. M. Shisslak, M. Crago, and L. S. Estes, "The Spectrum of Eating Disturbances," *International Journal of Eating Disorders* 18, no. 3 (November 1995): 209–19.

12. Natalia Zunino, PhD, of American Anorexia and Bulimia Association, Inc. in "Eating Disorder Statistics," The Alliance for Eating Disorders Awareness, ndsu.edu/fileadmin/counseling/Eating_Disorder_Statistics.pdf.

13. M. J. De Souza, A. Nattiv, E. Joy, et al., "2014 Female Athlete Triad Coalition Consensus Statement on Treatment and Return to Play of the Female Athlete Triad, 1st International Conference held in San Francisco, CA, May 2012, and 2nd International Conference held in Indianapolis, IN, May 2013," *Clinical Journal of Sport Medicine* 24, no. 2 (March 2014): 96–119.

R. J. Mallinson, N. I. Williams, M. P. Olmsted, J. L. Scheid, E. S. Riddle, and M. J. De Souza, "A Case Report of Recovery of Menstrual Function Following a Nutritional Intervention in Two Exercising Women with Amenorrhea of Varying Duration," *Journal of the International Society of Sports Nutrition* 10 (August 2013): 34.

14. C. Laird Birmingham, J. V. Pierre, *Beumont Medical Management of Eating Disorders: A Practical Handbook for Healthcare Providers*, (Cambridge: Cambridge University Press, 2010).

15. J. Yager, M. J. Devlin, K. A. Halmi, et al., "Practice Guideline for the Treatment of Patients with Eating Disorders," 3rd Ed., (Washington, DC: American Psychiatric Association, 2010).

16. D. W. Garner, S. C. Wooley, "Confronting the Failure of Behavioral and Dietary Treatments for Obesity," *Clinical Psychology Review* 11, no. 6 (1991): 727–80.

Chapter 2: Family-Based Treatment (FBT)

1. J. Lock and D. Le Grange, *Treatment Manual for Anorexia Nervosa: A Family-Based Approach*, 2nd ed. (New York: Guilford, 2013).

   J. Lock, "Evaluation of Family Treatment Models for Eating Disorders" *Current Opinion in Psychiatry* 24, no. 4 (July 2011), 274–79.

2. J. Lock and D. Le Grange, "Family-Based Treatment of Eating Disorders," *International Journal of Eating Disorders* 37, supplement (2005): 64–67.

3. I. Eisler, C. Dare, G. F. M. Russell, G. I. Szmukler, D. Le Grange, and E. Dodge, "Family and Individual Therapy in Anorexia Nervosa: A Five-Year Follow-up," *Archives of General Psychiatry* 54, no. 11 (November 1997): 1025–30.

4. D. Le Grange, J. Lock, W. S. Agras, S. W. Bryson, B. Jo, "Randomized Clinical Trial of Family-Based Treatment and Cognitive-Behavioral Therapy for Adolescent Bulimia Nervosa," *Journal of the American Academy of Child and Adolescent Psychiatry, US National Library of Medicine* 54, no. 11 (November 2015): 886–94.

5. June Alexander and Daniel Le Grange, *My Kid Is Back: Empowering Parents to Beat Anorexia Nervosa* (New York City: Routledge, 2009).

6. A. Smith, C. Cook-Cottone, "A Review of Family Therapy as an Effective Intervention for Anorexia Nervosa in Adolescents," *Journal of Clinical Psychology Medical Settings* 18, no. 4 (October 2011): 323–34.

7. P. Doyle, D. Le Grange, K. Loeb, et al., "Early response to family-based treatment for adolescent anorexia nervosa." *International Journal of Eating Disorders* 43, no. 7 (November 2010): 659–62.

8. D. Le Grange, J. Lock, W. S. Agras, A. Moye, S. W. Bryson, B. Jo, H. C. Kraemer, "Predictors of Drop Out and Remission in FBT," *International Journal of Eating Disorders* volume 50, no. 2 (December 2006): 85–92.

9. D. Le Grange et al., "Predictors and Moderators of Outcome in FBT for Adolescents with Bulimia Nervosa," *Journal of the American Academy of Child and Adolescent Psychiatry* 47, no. 4 (April 2008): pages 464–70.

    D. Le Grange, J. Lock, et al., "Moderators and Mediators of Remission in Family-Based Treatment and Adolescent Focused Therapy for Anorexia Nervosa," *Behaviour Research and Therapy* 50, no. 2 (February 2012): 85–92.

10. J. Lock, et al., "Randomized Clinical Trial Comparing FBT with AFT for Adolescents with Anorexia Nervosa," *Archives of General Psychiatry* volume 67, no. 10 (October 2010): 1025–32.

11. J. Lock and D. Le Grange, *Treatment Manual for Anorexia Nervosa*.

12. Eva Musby, *Anorexia and Other Eating Disorders: How to Help Your Child Eat Well and Be Well: Practical Solutions, Compassionate Communication Tools and Emotional Support for Parents of Children and Teenagers*, (APRICA, 2014).

13. Maria Ganci, *Survive FBT: Skills Manual for Parents Undertaking Family Based Treatment (FBT) for Child and Adolescent Anorexia Nervosa* (Melbourne: LMD Publishing, 2016).

14. R. Ellison, P. Rhodes, S. Madden, J. Miskovic, A. Wallis, A. Baillie, M. Kohn, S. Touyz, "Do the Components of Manualized Family-Based Treatment for Anorexia Nervosa Predict Weight Gain?" *International Journal of Eating Disorders* 45, no. 4 (May 2012): 609–14.

15. J. Lock and D. Le Grange, *Treatment Manual for Anorexia Nervosa*, 123–24.

16. Joanna Elise Wiese, "A Qualitative Analysis of Parental Experiences in Family-Based Treatment for Anorexia Nervosa," PhD thesis, University of Iowa, 2014, ir.uiowa.edu/etd/1515.

Chapter 3: It Takes a Village: Getting Help from Your Team

1. J. Arcelus, A. Mitchell, J. Wales, et al., "Mortality Rates in Patients with Anorexia Nervosa and Other Eating Disorders: A Meta-Analysis of 36 Studies," *Archives of General Psychiatry* 68, no. 7 (July 2011): 724–31, doi:10.1001/archgenpsychiatry.2011.74.

Chapter 4: Common Medical Issues

1. N. H. Golden, D. K. Katzman, S. M. Sawyer, R. M. Ornstein, E. S. Rome, A. K. Garber, M. Kohn, R. E. Kreipe, "Position Paper of the Society for Adolescent Health and Medicine: Medical Management of Restrictive Eating Disorders in Adolescents and Young Adults," *Journal of Adolescent Health* 56, no. 1 (January 2015): 121–25, doi:10.1016/j.jadohealth.2014.10.259.

2. J. Couturier, L. Isserlin, and J.Lock, "Family-Based Treatment for Adolescents With Anorexia Nervosa: A Dissemination Study," *Eating Disorders* 18, no. 3 (May 2010): 199–209.

3. M. R. Kohn, N. H. Golden, and I. R. Shenker. "Cardiac Arrest and Delirium: Presentations of the Refeeding Syndrome in Severely Malnourished Adolescents with Anorexia Nervosa," *Journal of Adolescent Health* 22, no. 3 (March 1998): 239–43.

4. R. M. Ornstein, N. H. Golden, M. S. Jacobson, and I. R. Shenker, "Hypophosphatemia During Nutritional Rehabilitation in Anorexia Nervosa: Implications for Refeeding and Monitoring," *Journal of Adolescent Health* 32, no. 1 (January 2003): 83–88.

   S. M. Solomon and D. F. Kirby, "The Refeeding Syndrome: A Review," *Journal of Parenteral and Enteral Nutrition* 14, no. 1 (January–February 1990): 90–97.

5. C. L. Tseng, O. Soroka, M. Maney, D. C. Aron, L. M. Pogach, "Assessing Potential Glycemic Overtreatment in Persons at Hypoglycemic Risk," *JAMA Internal Medicine* 174, no. 2 (February 2014): 259–68.

6. R. W. Smith, C. Korenblum, K. Thacker K, H. J. Bonifacio, T. Gonska, and D. K. Katzman, "Severely Elevated Transaminases in an Adolescent Male with Anorexia Nervosa," *International Journal of Eating Disorders* 46, no. 7 (November 2013): 751–54.

7. Richard Nyeko, et al., "Lactose Intolerance Among Severely Malnourished Children with Diarrhoea Admitted to the Nutrition Unit, Mulago Hospital, Uganda," *BMC Pediatrics* 10, no. 1 (June 2010): 31, doi:10.1186/1471-2431-10-31.

8. R. Dalle-Grave, S. Calugi, and G. Marchesini, "Is Amenorrhea a Useful Criterion for the Diagnosis of Anorexia Nervosa?," *Behaviour Research and Therapy* 46, no. 12 (December 2008): 1290–96.

9. The Practice Committee of the American Society for Reproductive Medicine, "Current Evaluation of Amenorrhea," *Fertility and Sterility* 86, no. 5 (November 2006): 148–55, doi:10.1016/j.fertnstert.2006.08.013.

10. N. Micali, I. Dos Santos Silva, B. De Stavola, et al., "Fertility Treatment, Twin Births, and Unplanned Pregnancies in Women with Eating Disorders: Findings from a Population-Based Birth Cohort." *BJOG: An International Journal of Obstetrics and Gynaecology* 121, no. 4 (March 2014): 408–16.

11. A. M. Miller, "The Lasting Toll of an Eating Disorder," *U.S. News and World Report*, March 31, 2016, health.usnews.com/wellness/articles/2016-03-31/the-lasting-toll-of-an-eating-disorder-fertility-issues.

12. N. H. Golden, M. S. Jacobson, J. Schebendach, et al., "Resumption of Menses in Anorexia Nervosa," *Archives of Pediatrics and Adolescent Medicine* 151, no. 1 (January 1997):16–21.

13. N. H. Golden, et al. "Treatment Goal Weight in Adolescents with Anorexia Nervosa: Use of BMI Percentiles," *International Journal of Eating Disorders* 41, no. 4 (May 2008): 301–6, doi:10.1002/eat.20503

14. Wendy Meyer Sterling, et al., "Metabolic Assessment of Menstruating and Nonmenstruating Normal Weight Adolescents," *International Journal of Eating Disorders* 42, no. 7 (November 2009): 658–63, doi:10.1002/eat.20604.

15. A. Nadjarzadeh, R. D. Firouzabadi, N. Vaziri, et al., "The Effect of Omega-3 Supplementation on Androgen Profile and Menstrual Status in Women with Polycystic Ovary Syndrome: A Randomized Clinical Trial," *Iranian Journal of Reproductive Medicine* 11, no. 8 (August 2013): 665–72.

16. "Choose Healthy Fats," Academy of Nutrition and Dietetics, March 6, 2017, eatright.org/resource/food/nutrition/dietary-guidelines-and-myplate/choose-healthy-fats.

17. S. Naessen, K. Carlstrom, R. Glant, et al., "Bone Mineral Density in Bulimic Women Influence of Endocrine Factors and Previous Anorexia," *European Journal of Endocrinology* 155, no. 2 (August 2006): 245–51.

18. S. Grinspoon, E. Thomas, S. Pitts, et al., "Prevalence and Predictive Factors for Regional Osteopenia in Women with Anorexia Nervosa," *Annals of Internal Medicine* 133 (November 2000): 790–94.

19. N. A. Rigotti, R. M. Neer, S. J. Skates, et al., "The Clinical Course of Osteoporosis in Anorexia Nervosa. A Longitudinal Study of Cortical Bone Mass," *JAMA* 265, no. 9 (March 1991): 1133–38.

20. L. K. Bachrach, D. K. Katzman, I. F. Litt, et al., "Recovery from Osteopenia in Adolescent Girls with Anorexia Nervosa," *Journal of Clinical Endocrinology and Metabolism* 72, no. 3 (March 1991): 602–6.

N. H. Golden, L. Lanzkowsky, J. Schebendach, et al., "The Effect of Estrogen-progestin Treatment on Bone Mineral Density in Anorexia Nervosa," *Journal of Pediatric and Adolescent Gynecology* 15, no. 3 (August 2002): 135–43.

21. P. K. Fazeli and A. Klibanski, "Bone Metabolism in Anorexia Nervosa," *Current Osteoporosis Reports* 12, no. 1 (March 2014): 82–89.

22. N. H. Golden, et al., "Effect of Estrogen-progestin Treatment."

23. Ibid.

24. J. J. Kraeft, R. N. Uppot, and A. M. Heffess, "Imaging Findings in Eating Disorders," *AJR American Journal of Roentgenology* 200, no. 4 (April 2013): W328–35.

25. M. Feldman and I. Meyer, "Eating Disorders in Diverse, Lesbian, Gay, and Bisexual Populations," *International Journal of Eating Disorders* 40, no. 3 (November 2007): 218–26.

26. J. Schebendach, N. H. Golden, M. S. Jacobson, et al., "Indirect Calorimetry in the Nutritional Management of Eating Disorders," *International Journal of Eating Disorders* 17, no. 1 (January 1995): 59–66.

N. Vaisman, M. F. Rossi, E. Goldberg, et al., "Energy Expenditure and Body Composition in Patients with Anorexia Nervosa," *Journal of Pediatrics* 113 (1988): 919–24.

27. J. E. Schebendach, N. H. Golden, M. S. Jacobson, et al., "The Metabolic Responses to Starvation and Refeeding in Adolescents with Anorexia Nervosa" *Annals of the New York Academy of Sciences* 817, (May 1997): 110–19.

N. Vaisman, M. F. Rossi, M. Corey, R. Clarke, E. Goldberg, and P. B. Pencharz, "Effect of Refeeding on the Energy Metabolism of Adolescent Girls Who Have Anorexia Nervosa," *European Journal of Clinical Nutrition* 45, no. 11 (November 1991): 527–37.

28. N. H. Golden and W. Meyer, "Nutritional Rehabilitation of Anorexia Nervosa. Goals and Dangers," *International Journal of Adolescent Medicine and Health* 16, no. 2 (April–June 2004): pages 131–44, doi:10.1515/ijamh.2004.16.2.131.

29. N. H. Golden, D. K. Katzman, S. M. Sawyer, et al., "Position Paper of the Society for Adolescent Health and Medicine: Medical Management of Restrictive Eating Disorders in Adolescents and Young Adults," *Journal of Adolescent Health* 56, no. 1 (January 2015): 121–25, doi:10.1016/j.jadohealth.2014.10.259.

Chapter 5: To Exercise or Not: Managing Athletes, Exercise, and Compulsive Movement

1. M. Freimuth, S. Moniz, and S. R. Kim, "Clarifying Exercise Addiction: Differential Diagnosis, Co-occurring Disorders, and Phases of Addiction," *International Journal of Environmental Research and Public Health* 8, no. 10 (October 2011): 4069–81.

2. J. Sundgot-Borgen and M. Klungland Torstveit, "Prevalence of Eating Disorders in Elite Athletes Is Higher Than in the General Population," *Clinical Journal of Sport Medicine* 14, no. 1 (January 2004): 25–32.

3. M. Mountjoy, J. Sundgot-Borgen, L. Burke, et al., "The IOC consensus statement: beyond the Female Athlete Triad—Relative Energy Deficiency in Sports (RED-S)." *British Journal of Sports Medicine* 48, no. 7 (April 2014): 491–97, doi:10.1136/bjsports-2014-093502.

4. D. E. Greydanus, H. Omar, H.D. Pratt, "The Adolescent Female Athlete: Current Concepts and Conundrums," *Pediatric Clinics of North America* 57, no. 3 (June 2010): 697–718, doi:10.1016/j.pcl.2010.02.005.

5. A. Dueck, K. S. Matt, M. M. Manore, et al., "Treatment of Athletic Amenorrhea with a Diet and Training Intervention Program," *International Journal of Sport Nutrition and Exercise* 6, no. 1 (March 1996): 24–40.

   C. P. Guebels, L. C. Kam, G. F. Maddalozzo, et al., "Active Women Before/ After an Intervention Designed to Restore Menstrual Function: Resting Metabolic Rate and Comparison of Four Methods to Quantify Energy Expenditure and Energy Availability," *International Journal of Sport Nutrition and Exercise Metabolism* 24, no. 1 (February 2014): 37–46.

   S. A. Kopp-Woodroffe, M. M. Manore, C. A. Dueck, et al., "Energy and Nutrient Status of Amenorrheic Athletes Participating in a Diet and Exercise Training Intervention Program," *International Journal of Sport Nutrition and Exercise* 9, no. 1 (March 1999): 70–88.

6. M. Freimuth, et al., "Clarifying Exercise Addiction."

7. C. M. Bonci, et al., "National Athletic Trainers' Association Position Statement: Preventing, Detecting, and Managing Disordered Eating in Athletes," *Journal of Athletic Training* 43, no. 1 (January–March 2008): 80–108, doi:10.4085/1062-6050-43.1.80.

Chapter 7: The Plate-by-Plate Approach: Making Sure Your Child Gets Enough Food

1. N. H. Golden, et al., "Higher Caloric Intake in Hospitalized Adolescents with Anorexia Nervosa Is Associated with Reduced Length of Stay and No Increased Rate of Refeeding Syndrome," *Journal of Adolescent Health* 53, no. 5 (November 2013): 573–78.

2. S. F. Forman, L. F. Grodin, D. A. Graham, et al., "An Eleven Site National Quality Improvement Evaluation of Adolescent Medicine-Based Eating Disorder Programs: Predictors of Weight Outcomes at One year and Risk Adjustment Analyses," *Journal of Adolescent Health* 49, no. 6 (December 2011): 594–600.

3. R. Duyff, "How Many Calories Does My Teen Need?" Academy of Nutrition and Dietetics, September 26, 2017, eatright.org/resource/food/nutrition/dietary-guidelines-and-myplate/how-many-calories-does-my-teen-need.

Chapter 8: Why This Breakdown? A Close-up on Grains/Starches, Proteins, Fruits and Vegetables, Fats, and Dairy

1. "A Teenager's Nutritional Needs," American Academy of Pediatrics, last modified March 1, 2016, healthychildren.org/English/ages-stages/teen/nutrition/Pages/A-Teenagers-Nutritional-Needs.aspx.

2. J. Castle, "How Teen Athletes Can Build Muscle with Protein," Academy of Nutrition and Dietetics, June 24, 2015, eatright.org/resource/fitness/sports-and-performance/fueling-your-workout/how-teen-athletes-can-build-muscles-with-protein.

3. "How Much Calcium Do Children and Teens Need?" US Department of Health and Human Services, last modified December 1, 2016, nichd.nih.gov/health/topics/bonehealth/conditioninfo/Pages/children.aspx.

Chapter 10: What to Do If Your Child Still Isn't Gaining Enough Weight: Accelerated Nutritional Rehabilitation

1. J. E. Schebendach, N. H. Golden, M. S. Jacobson, et al., "The Metabolic Responses to Starvation and Refeeding in Adolescents with Anorexia Nervosa," *Annals of the New York Academy of Sciences* 817 (May 1997): 110–19.

2. N. H. Golden and W. Meyer, "Nutritional Rehabilitation of Anorexia Nervosa."

3. N. H. Golden, "Higher Caloric Intake in Hospitalized Adolescents."

   D. Le Grange, et al., "Early Weight Gain Predicts Outcome in Two Treatments for Adolescent Anorexia Nervosa."

4. "Tips on Controlling Gas," International Foundation for Functional Gastrointestinal Disorders, last modified September 18, 2015, iffgd.org/symptoms-causes/intestinal-gas/tips-on-controlling-gas.html.

Chapter 12: How to Talk About Diet and Weight (Hint: Don't!)

1. "Dinner Games," The Family Dinner Project, thefamilydinnerproject.org/fun/dinner-games.

Chapter 14: Moving Beyond Brown Rice: Letting Go of Food Fears

1. L. L. Birch, et al., "What Kind of Exposure Reduces Children's Food Neophobia?" *Appetite* 9, no. 3 (December 1987): 171–78, doi:10.1016/s0195-6663(87)80011-9.

   L. L. Birch and D. W. Marlin, "I Don't Like It; I Never Tried It: Effects of Exposure on Two-Year-Old Children's Food Preferences," *Appetite* 3, no. 4 (December 1982), 353–60, doi:10.1016/s0195-6663(82)80053-6.

2. K. Tchanturia, H. Davies, C. Reeder, et al., *Cognitive Remediation Therapy for Anorexia Nervosa*, (London 2010), national.slam.nhs.uk/wp-content/uploads/2014/04/Cognitive-remediation-therapy-for-Anorexia-Nervosa-Kate-Tchantura.pdf.

3. C. L. Dahlgren, B. Lask, N. I. Landrø, and Ø. Rø, "Developing and Evaluating Cognitive Remediation Therapy (CRT) for Adolescents with Anorexia Nervosa: A Feasibility Study," *Clinical Child Psychology and Psychiatry* 19, no. 3 (July 2014): 476–87.

   K. Tchanturia, N. Lounes, and S. Holttum, "Cognitive Remediation in Anorexia Nervosa and Related Conditions: A Systematic Review," *European Eating Disorders Review* 22, no. 6 (November 2014): 454–62.

   B. M. van Noort, M. K. A. Kraus, E. Pfeiffer, U. Lehmkuhl, and V. Kappel, "Neuropsychological and Behavioural Short-Term Effects of Cognitive Remediation Therapy in Adolescent Anorexia Nervosa: A Pilot Study," *European Eating Disorders Review* 24, no. 1 (January 2016): 69–74.

4. Dahlgren, C. L., van Noort, B., Lask B., "The Cognitive Remediation Therapy (CRT) Resource Pack for Children and Adolescents with Feeding and Eating Disorders," 2nd ed. (Oslo: Oslo University Hospital, 2015), doi:10.13140/RG.2.1.1279.5364.

5. "The Importance of Family Dinners VIII," The National Center on Addiction and Substance Abuse, September 2012, centeronaddiction.org/addiction-research/reports/importance-of-family-dinners-2012.

Chapter 15: Returning to Normal (Phase 3 of FBT)

1. E. Satter, "What Is Normal Eating?" Ellyn Satter Institute, 2018, ellynsatterinstitute.org/wp-content/uploads/2017/11/What-is-normal-eating-Secure.pdf.

2. N. H. Golden et al., "Resumption of Menses."

3. E. Satter, "Adult Eating and Weight," Ellyn Satter Institute, 2018, ellynsatterinstitute.org/how-to-eat/adult-eating-and-weight.

FURTHER READING

Books for Parents

Brown, Harriet, and Daniel Le Grange. *Brave Girl Eating: A Family's Struggle with Anorexia.* New York: Harper, 2011.

Ganci, Maria. *Survive FBT: Skills Manual for Parents Undertaking Family Based Treatment (FBT) for Child and Adolescent Anorexia Nervosa.* Melbourne: LMD, 2016.

Herrin, Marcia, and Nancy Matsumoto. *The Parent's Guide to Eating Disorders: Supporting Self-esteem, Healthy Eating, and Positive Body Image at Home.* Carlsbad, CA: Gurze, 2007.

Kater, Kathy. *Real Kids Come in All Sizes: Ten Essential Lessons to Build Your Child's Body Esteem.* New York: Broadway, 2004.

Lock, James, and Daniel Le Grange. *Help Your Teenager Beat an Eating Disorder*, 2nd ed. New York: Guilford, 2015.

Musby, Eva. *Anorexia and Other Eating Disorders: How to Help Your Child Eat Well and Be Well.* Aprica, 2014.

Neumark-Sztainer, Dianne. *"I'm, Like, SO Fat!": Helping Your Teen Make Healthy Choices about Eating and Exercise in a Weight-Obsessed World.* New York: Guilford, 2005.

Norton, Claire P. *Feeding Your Anorexic Adolescent.* Nutripress, 2009.

Satter, Ellyn. *Secrets of Feeding a Healthy Family: How to Eat, How to Raise Good Eaters, How to Cook.* Madison, WI: Kelcy, 2008.

Books for Individuals in Recovery

Fairburn, Christopher G. *Overcoming Binge Eating: The Proven Program to Learn Why You Binge and How You Can Stop.* New York: Guilford, 2013.

Heffner, Michelle, Georg H. Eifert, and Steven C. Hayes. *The Anorexia Workbook: How to Accept Yourself, Heal Your Suffering, and Reclaim Your Life.* Oakland, CA: New Harbinger, 2004.

Koenig, Kathy. *Rules of "Normal" Eating: A Commonsense Approach for Dieters, Overeaters, Undereaters, Emotional Eaters, and Everyone in Between.* Carlsbad, CA: Gurze, 2005.

LoBue, Andrea, and Marsea Marcus. *The Don't Diet, Live-it! Workbook: Healing Food, Weight and Body Issues.* Carlsbad, CA: Gurze, 1999.

McCabe, Randi E., Traci L. McFarlane, and Marion P. Olmsted. *The Overcoming Bulimia Workbook: Your Comprehensive, Step-by-Step Guide to Recovery.* Oakland, CA: New Harbinger, 2004.

Schaefer, Jenni, and Thom Rutledge. *Life without Ed.* New York: McGraw-Hill Education, 2014. (To help understand all the thinking that goes on with someone with an eating disorder.)

Thomas, Jennifer J., and Jenni Schaefer. *Almost Anorexic: Is My (or My Loved One's) Relationship with Food a Problem?* Center City, MN: Hazelden, 2013.

Walen, Andrew. *Man Up to Eating Disorders.* Cork: BookBaby, 2014.

Body-Positive Health Books

Bacon, Linda. *Health at Every Size: The Surprising Truth about Your Weight*, Dallas, TX: BenBella Books, 2010.

Bacon, Linda, and Lucy Aphramor. *Body Respect: What Conventional Health Books Get Wrong, Leave Out, and Just Plain Fail to Understand about Weight.* Dallas, TX: BenBella Books, 2014.

Body-Positivity Books for Children

Haduch, Bill, and Rick Stromoski. *Food Rules!: The Stuff You Munch, Its Crunch, Its Punch, and Why You Sometimes Lose Your Lunch.* New York: Puffin, 2001. (This illustrated book is for kids aged nine to fourteen.)

Mills, Andy, Becky Osborn, and Erica Neitz. *Shapesville.* Carlsbad, CA: Gurze, 2003. (This illustrated book is for kids aged three to eight.)

EDUCATIONAL AND NONPROFIT ORGANIZATIONS

United States

About Face

Website: about-face.org

Dedicated to educating women about harmful media messages that affect their self-esteem and body image

Academy for Eating Disorders

Phone: 703-234-4079

Website: aedweb.org

Provides resources for professionals, students, and patients

Academy of Nutrition and Dietetics

Website: eatright.org

Offers an extensive nutrition reading list and database of dietitians specializing in eating disorders

Alliance for Eating Disorders Awareness

Phone: 561-841-0900

Website: allianceforeatingdisorders.com

Provides educational materials to parents and caregivers

Binge Eating Disorder Association (BEDA)

Website: bedaonline.com

Focuses on recognition, prevention, and treatment of BED and associated weight stigma; provides a long list of further resources and a referral link to providers

The Body Positive

Phone: 510.528.0101

Email: info@thebodypositive.org

Website: thebodypositive.org

Promotes body positive programs among teens and young adults

Diabulimia Helpline

Twenty-four-hour hotline: 425-985-3635

Dedicated to education, support, and advocacy for diabetics with eating disorders, and their loved ones

Eating Disorder Hope

Website: eatingdisorderhope.com

Connects sufferers to others in recovery in search of hope, health, and healing

Eating Disorder Referral and Information Center

Website: edreferral.com

Provides referrals to eating disorder professionals, treatment facilities, and support groups

Families Empowered and Supporting Treatment of Eating Disorders (FEAST)

Website: feast-ed.org

Provides individual listings and educational information about eating disorders

Maudsley Parents

Website: maudsleyparents.org

Provides individual listings for providers who specialize in family-based treatment/the Maudsley approach

Mirror Mirror

Website: mirror-mirror.org

Provides information, education, and support to the community, including people dealing with eating disorders and information for their caregivers

National Association for Males with Eating Disorders (NAMED)

Website: namedinc.org

Provides support for men with eating disorders

National Association of Anorexia Nervosa and Associated Disorders

Helpline: 630-577-1330

Email: anadhelp@anad.org

Website: anad.org

Hotline counseling and a national network of free support groups, referrals to treatment specialists, and programs to boost self-acceptance

National Eating Disorders Association

Website: nationaleatingdisorders.org

Helpline: 800-931-2237

Supports individuals and families affected by eating disorders and provides treatment referrals

Project HEAL

Website: theprojectheal.org

Nonprofit that provides funding for the treatment of eating disorders, as well as a peer mentorship program, outreach, and education in the community

Something Fishy

Website: something-fishy.org

Dedicated to raising awareness with bulletin boards, online chats, and referrals

Canada

ANEB (Anorexia and Bulimia Quebec)

514-630-0907

Website: anebquebec.com

Bulimia Anorexia Nervosa Association

Website: bana.ca

Eating Disorders Foundation of Canada

Website: edfofcanada.com

Supports local community groups

Hope's Eating Disorders Support

Phone: 519-434-7721

Website: hopeseds.org

Provides a library, support groups, educational workshops, outreach, information, drop-in support, and referral about treatment centers, therapists, and nutritionists

Hopewell/Eating Disorders Support Centre of Ottawa

Phone: 613-241-3428

Website: hopewell.ca

Provides eating-disorder resources and support for treatment and recovery

Jessie's Legacy

Website: jessieslegacy.com

A program of Family Services of the North Shore; a community-based agency that offers education, support, and counseling services

Kelty Eating Disorders

Phone: 604-875-2084, or toll-free from anywhere in British Columbia: 1-800-665-1822

Email: keltycentre@cw.bc.ca

Website: keltyeatingdisorders.ca

Provides mental-health and substance-use information, resources, help with system navigation, and peer support to children, youth, and their families from across British Columbia

Looking Glass Foundation

Phone: 604-314-0548

Email: info@lookingglassbc.com

Website: lookingglassbc.com

Helps with early intervention and programs for eating-disorder support, recovery, and sustained relapse prevention

National Eating Disorder Information Centre

Phone: 866-NEDIC-20 (toll-free) or 416-340-4156

Email: nedic@uhn.on.ca

Website: nedic.ca

Provides information and resources for the treatment of eating disorders

Sheena's Place

Phone: 416-927-8900

Website: sheenasplace.org

Sheena's Place, located in downtown Toronto, offers group support for individuals seventeen years of age and older struggling with eating disorders, as well as support for family, friends, and partners who have a loved one struggling with an eating disorder. Individuals do not require a referral or a diagnosis to attend groups at Sheena's Place. All groups at Sheena's Place are offered free of charge.

Australia

Bridges Eating Disorder Association

Website: bridges.net.au

Provides support services for all people affected by eating disorders in Western Australia

Butterfly Foundation

National Helpline 1800 33 4673, Monday to Friday 8:00 a.m. to 9:00 p.m. AEST

Website: thebutterflyfoundation.org.au

Provides direct financial relief, advocacy, awareness campaigns, health promotion, and early intervention work

Centre for Eating & Dieting Disorders (CEDD)

Website: cedd.org.au

A service-development, research, and clinical excellence center that engages in large-scale service development projects, workforce-training programs, and research projects

Eating Disorders Association, Inc. (Queensland)

Website: eda.org.au

Provides eating-disorder information and referrals, individual and family counseling, group support, peer support, education, and skills-based training to caregivers

Eating Disorders Victoria

Phone: 1300 550 236

Email: help@eatingdisorders.org.au

Website: eatingdisorders.org.au

A comprehensive source of reliable and factual information on eating disorders. Provides a helpline, private psychology sessions, a peer-mentoring program, and support groups

National Eating Disorders Collaboration (NEDC)

National Helpline: 1800 33 4673

Phone: 02 9412 4499

Fax: 02 8090 8196

Email: info@nedc.com.au

Website: nedc.com.au

Provides information, resources, and access to professionals for those affected by an eating disorder and promotes community awareness for eating disorder prevention

Ireland

Bodywhys: The Eating Disorders Association of Ireland

Website: bodywhys.ie

New Zealand

Canterbury Mental Health Education and Resource Centre

Phone: 03 365 5344

Website: mherc.org.nz

Provides information, resources, and support groups

Eating Disorder Associate of New Zealand (EDANZ)

Phone: 0800 2 EDANZ

Email: info@ed.org.nz

Website: ed.org.nz

Provides support, education, and awareness for caretakers of people with eating disorders

United Kingdom

Beat Eating Disorders

Phone: 0300 123 3355

Email: info@beateatingdisorders.org.uk

Website: beateatingdisorders.org.uk

The UK's eating-disorder charity. Provides helplines, online support groups, message boards, and access to professional help for anyone affected by an eating disorder

Help for adults

The **Beat Adult Helpline** is open to anyone over eighteen. Parents, teachers, or any concerned adults should call the adult helpline.

Helpline: 0808 801 0677

Email: help@beateatingdisorders.org.uk

Help for adolescents

The **Beat Youthline** is open to anyone under eighteen.

Youthline: 0808 801 0711

Email: fyp@beateatingdisorders.org.uk

Men Get Eating Disorders Too (MGEDT)

Website: mengetedstoo.co.uk

Raises awareness of eating disorders in men and provides support for sufferers, caregivers, and their families

National Centre for Eating Disorders

Phone: +44 (0)845 838 2040

Fax: +44 (0)1372 469550

Website: eating-disorders.org.uk

Provides information about eating disorders and lists of professionals in local areas

Somerset and Wessex Eating Disorders Association

Phone: 01749 34 33 44

Email: support@swedauk.org

Website: swedauk.org

Provides counseling, a monthly self-help support group, and a college support service

Additional Resources

The Dad Man

Website: joekelly.org

Eating Disorder Family Support

Website: eatingdisorderfamilysupport.com

Health at Every Size

Website: haescommunity.com

ACKNOWLEDGMENTS

We would like to acknowledge those who have helped us cultivate this approach along the way. First, to the Healthy Teen Project, who believed in our innovation, and encouraged us to implement the Plate-by-Plate Approach so that it could fully develop. We would like to thank James Lock, MD, PhD, director of the Eating Disorder Program at Lucile Packard Children's Hospital at Stanford, for his heartfelt foreword supporting our approach and his guidance along the way. We would like to thank Neville H. Golden, MD, chief of Adolescent Medicine at Lucile Packard Children's Hospital at Stanford, for his beautifully written foreword and for his expert review of chapter 4. To the Adolescent Eating Disorders team at Lucile Packard Children's Hospital at Stanford for your allegiance and contributions to family-based treatment upon which we have built the principles of this approach. We would like to thank Dr. Daniel LeGrange, director of psychiatry at UCSF, for allowing us to share our approach with his team and for his support and feedback. To Susanne Martin, MD, for her medical expertise, passion for this work, and tireless review of the medical chapter; Nan Shaw, LCSW, for her beautiful way with words, wise counsel, friendship, and her mastery of FBT showcased in chapter 2, which we know will make the FBT community proud. To Rollyn Ornstein, MD, professor of pediatrics at the Penn State College of Medicine in the Division of Adolescent Medicine and Eating Disorders at Penn State Hershey Children's Hospital, we are grateful for your expert and careful review of chapter 4. Riley Nickols, PhD, sport psychologist at the Victory Program for his guidance on physical activity in the eating disorder population, and his assistance with chapter 5 and chapter 11; Nick Paparesta, head trainer at the Oakland A's for his expertise on recovery and rest; Elizabeth Scott, LCSW, cofounder of the Body Positive, for allowing us to share her wisdom in chapter 12; Camilla Lindvall Dahlgren, PhD, senior researcher at the Regional Department for Eating Disorders, Oslo University Hospital, for allowing us to pick her brain on cognitive remediation therapy used in the treatment of eating disorders as found in chapter 14; Liana Rosenman, cofounder of Project HEAL, for her inspiring words about recovery and body image; and Carrie Spindel, PsyD, for her guidance and expertise on exposure.

To our own "village" of professionals we have worked with over the years, we have learned so much from you and continue to every day. We admire your heart, your fervor, and your dedication to treating and *beating* eating disorders, these kids truly get better because of you. And lastly, to all of the teens and families we have worked with over the years, thank you for trusting us with your care; we have been honored to be part of your journey and wish you all true freedom from this terrible illness.

We would be remiss if we didn't mention those who personally supported and encouraged us.

Casey: To Katie Bell, NP, and Jennifer Zumarraga, MD, for your unwavering belief in my abilities, not only as a dietitian, but as a leader—thank you for pushing me in the direction of my dreams. To my incredible team at the Healthy Teen Project, because of you I don't ever "go to work," I live for it. You inspire me every single day and I am honored to be a part of this endeavor with you. I would like to personally thank Neville Golden, MD, Cynthia Kapphahn, MD, Lorraine Mulvihill, RD, Emily Wortiska, RD, and Kortney Parman, NP, RD, for entrusting me with the nutrition program at the Comprehensive Eating Disorders Program at Lucile Packard Children's Hospital right out of my internship. You saw a spark that I didn't even know I had and you shaped me into the dietitian I am today. To my dietetic internship class at UC Davis Medical Center, Alice Vasilev, MS, RD, CNSC, Katy Miller, RD, CNSC, Brittany Scaniello, RD, Peter Mak, RD, and Allison Reitz, MS, RD, I'm beyond lucky to have walked that year beside you and I admire your contributions to the field. To Katie Di Lauro, RD, and Samantha Lalush, RD—you were the very best study partners and friends at Cal Poly and I'm so proud to know you.

To my loving family—my parents, Eileen Keane and Dave Miller, for setting the dinner table every single night with not only delicious food, but love. You knew how important it was to involve me in food, to teach me how to shop for, prepare, and *truly* enjoy food. And you taught me how to share that love for food with the world. The teens and families that I work with learn from YOU every single day. Thank you for teaching me what no one else could have, the true appreciation of food, a rare gem in this world of diet culture that I am beyond grateful to have. To my sisters (and best friends), Devon Anderson and Shannon Crossman, thank you for your unconditional love and support throughout our lifetime. You are incredibly talented women and I am in awe of the professionals, wives, and mothers you have become. And of course, to my loving husband, Ryan Crosbie. You have never stopped believing in me. Your support and your love through this process have been paramount in my ability to get through it. Your passion and drive for your own work inspires me to jump every hurdle without hesitation as I so often see you do. Thank you for your genuine curiosity about my work and for pushing me to never give up. And I cannot thank you enough for taking the time to put a delicious dinner on the table when I needed to write, for enthusiastically making every Sunday "Farmer's Market Day!" and for sharing in the true enjoyment of food that we will lovingly pass on to our future children. You and our baby-on-the-way have been incredibly patient, allowing me to write at odd hours and meet hectic deadlines throughout this pregnancy. I can't wait to see which arrives first, this book or our baby!

Wendy: I would like to personally thank my mentors and colleagues who have helped shape my way of evaluating and treating eating disorders and with whom I have closely collaborated over the years. First, I am grateful for getting the chance to learn from the best; the doctors, fellows, social workers, nurses, and psychiatrists at Cohen's Children's Hospital (formerly Schneider Children's Hospital at NS-LIJ), Division of Adolescent Medicine and Eating Disorders Center in New York led by Martin Fisher, MD, and the late Ronald I. Shenker, MD. Linda Filiberto,

RN, NPP, thank you for your mentorship and friendship, you were the first one to show me, through your amazing work, that these kids really do get better. I would like to especially thank Neville Golden, MD, for teaching me everything I know about adolescents and eating disorders, for his years of collaboration, mentorship, and friendship, both on the East Coast and West Coast. I would like to thank Katie Bell, NP, and Jennifer Zumarraga, MD, who invited me to join the Healthy Teen Project family; your commitment to families and their teens is amazing, and I am grateful for your close clinical collaboration and friendship. And Signe Darpinian, LMFT, for our daily calls and discussions about patients, writing books, and life.

To the sports organizations with which I have worked closely over the years—the Oakland Athletics, New York Jets, Golden State Warriors, and Menlo Athletics—thank you to the coaches, trainers, doctors, and psychologists that helped shape my expertise in sports. I am forever grateful for the opportunities to be part of the team and to work with such amazing and talented athletes.

To my closest friends from EBHS, Cornell, New York, and California, thank you for being by my side from the beginning, through long hours of studying, to grad school, to real life. I feel so lucky to have you all in my life. Thank you to my loving parents Fran and Stuart Meyer for insisting I get a good night's sleep and teaching me to love and embrace *all* foods, both of which I pass along to my clients and my daughters every day. Thank you for your encouragement to choose a career I love and for your unconditional love and support. To my sister, Bonnie Altman, thank you for allowing me to take the car to commute out to Long Island the year I started my career—I might have had an entirely different path otherwise! Thank you for your love, friendship, and advice over the years, I am forever grateful for the support from you, Matt, Jake, Evan, and Zachary. I would also like to thank my daughters, Emily and Lexi Sterling, for their sweet hugs and kisses, and for providing such good material for what "food freedom," found so naturally and innocently in children, really looks like. Lastly, to my husband, Peter Sterling, thank you for believing in me and reminding me that everything and anything is possible. Thank you for your love, friendship, patience, unwavering support, and all of the reminders to play more and work less.

And last but not least, we'd like to thank The Experiment for their belief in this project and interest in helping those struggling with eating disorders.

PERMISSIONS ACKNOWLEDGMENTS

INDEX

How to Nourish Your Child Through an Eating Disorder

How to Nourish Your Child Through an Eating Disorder

gastroparesis, 65–66
glucose, low, 62
gluten intolerance, 157
grains and starches, 124–26, 137, 153, 158
grocery shopping, 107

H

hair loss, 64
health messages, taking to extreme, 26
healthy approach to food, modeling, 192–94
Healthy Teen Project, 113–14
hematology, abnormal, 62–63
hidden calorie loss, 149–50
hormone levels, 67–73, 132–33
hospitalization, medical, 78, 79
"hugging the iceberg," 43
hunger cues, 252–53
hyperbilirubinemia, 65
hypermetabolism, 151
hypocarotenemia, 65, 131–32
hypoglycemia, 62
hypokalemia, 61
hypomagnesemia, 62
hyponatremia, 61
hypophosphatemia, 61
hypotension, orthostatic, 60

I

illness, 146
independence, introducing. *See* family-based treatment Phase 2
inner circle, 49–51
International Society for Clinical Densitometry, 72–73

Ireland organizations, 280
iron, 128–29

J

jaundice, 65
journals, food, 18

L

lactose intolerance, 157
Le Grange, Daniel, 33, 38
lipid panels, 63–64
liver transaminases, 62
Lock, James, 33, 34, 38
low glucose, 62
low magnesium, 62
low phosphorus, 61
low potassium, 61
low sodium, 61
lunch, 134, 136, 140, 156, 185
See also meal plans

M

magnesium, low, 62
malnutrition, assessing, 78, 80
Maudsley approach. 32
active, with added drinks, 170–71
active vegetarian, with added drinks, 172–73
standard plates, 162–63
standard plates, with added drinks, 166–67
standard vegetarian, 164–65
standard vegetarian, with added drinks, 168–69

nutritional needs of family
    members, 189–90
nutritional rehabilitation, as term,
    24

O

observing, 254–55
obsessive thinking, 17–19
oils, 71
oligomenorrhea, 17
omega-3 fatty acids, 69, 71
organizations, educational/
    nonprofit, 275–81
orthorexia, 22, 24–27, 231–33
orthostatic hypotension, 60
orthostatic tachycardia, 60
other specified feeding or eating
    disorder (OSFED), 13

P

Paparesta, Nick, 92
parents
    books for, 273
    fears, 195–96
    needs, explaining your, 194
    self-care, 56–57
    supervision of child at
        mealtime, 5, 111–12
    therapist for, 57
    worksheet, 240–42
    See also family members
pediatricians, 51, 52
perfectionism, 255
pericardial effusion, 59
phosphorus, low, 61
Plate-by-Plate approach
    about, 2–4

adjustments to plate, 155–56
breakfast, 139, 155
dinner, 141, 156
drinks, added, 155–56
family-based treatment and,
    44–45, 47–48
final review, 122–23
food groups, including all,
    117–19
foods, including variety of,
    121–22
gut, going with your, 147
lunch, 140, 156
meal examples and evaluations,
    139–42
meals and snacks, number of,
    121
MyPlate versus, 5–6
plate, filling up, 119–21
plate, size of, 116–17, 213
snacks, 143–45, 155, 156
special circumstances, 146
vegetarian plate, 142
plate size, 116–17, 213
portion sizes, restaurant, 207
post-workout meals, 21
potassium, low, 61
potatoes, sweet versus white,
    232–33
pregnancy, 69
primary amenorrhea, 77
professionals
    family-based therapists, 51, 53
    medical providers, 51, 52, 85
    psychiatrists, 52, 54
    recommendations from, 54
    registered dietitians, 52, 53
    united front with, 54

ABOUT THE AUTHORS

Casey Crosbie, RD, CSSD, is a specialist in adolescent eating disorders and currently serves as program director at the Healthy Teen Project, a partial hospitalization and intensive outpatient program for adolescents with eating disorders in Los Altos, California. She previously served as lead dietitian for the Lucile Packard Children's Hospital (LPCH) Comprehensive Care Program for Eating Disorders at Stanford. Casey was published in *Nutrition in Clinical Practice* (2012) and in the *Journal of Adolescent Health* (2013) for research focusing on refeeding syndrome as well as increased caloric intake and reduced length of hospitalization in adolescents with eating disorders. Casey received her BS in food science and nutrition from California Polytechnic State University, San Luis Obispo, and completed her dietetic internship at UC Davis Medical Center to earn her RD.

Wendy Sterling, MS, RD, CSSD, is an expert in adolescent nutrition, with a specialty in eating disorders and sports nutrition. Wendy is the team nutritionist for the Oakland Athletics and has previously consulted for the New York Jets and Golden State Warriors. Wendy has worked in the Eating Disorders Center at Cohen Children's Medical Center of New York and the Healthy Teen Project in Los Altos, California. She has conducted research on amenorrhea, metabolism, and osteoporosis which has been published in the *International Journal of Eating Disorders* and the *Journal of Adolescent Health*. Wendy is the coauthor of *No Weigh!! A Teen's Guide to Positive Body Image, Food, and Emotional Wisdom*. She received a BS in nutrition/dietetics from Cornell University and her MS/RD from Teachers College, Columbia University.

ABOUT THE CONTRIBUTORS

Dr. Susanne Martin is board certified in internal medicine and adolescent medicine. She is the medical director at the Healthy Teen Project and also works as a clinical instructor at Stanford's Vaden Health Center, Stanford School of Medicine, and at Sutter/Palo Alto Medical Foundation (PAMF) in urgent care. Dr. Martin is also the primary care provider for Center for Discovery, a residential treatment program in Menlo Park, California, that specializes in treating eating disorders in adolescents.

Nan Shaw is a licensed clinical social worker and FBT-credentialed therapist. She has been treating eating disorders for over thirty years, working in both inpatient and outpatient settings and specializing in treating both eating disorder sufferers and their families. In addition, Shaw held the position of best practices chair for eating disorders for Northern California Kaiser Permanente. She is currently in private practice in Los Altos, California.